14 95

DISCARDED

Winning the
Food Fight

D0150258

Winning the
Food Fight

How to Introduce Variety
into Your Child's Diet

NATALIE RIGAL

Translated by Jody Gladding

Healing Arts Press
Rochester, Vermont

Healing Arts Press
One Park Street
Rochester, Vermont 05767
www.HealingArtsPress.com

Healing Arts Press is a division of Inner Traditions International

Copyright © 2000 by Éditions Noesis
English translation copyright © 2006 by Inner Traditions International

Originally published in French under the title *La naissance du gout* by Éditions Noesis, Paris
First U.S. edition published in 2006 by Healing Arts Press

All rights reserved. No part of this book may be reproduced or utilized in any form or by any means, electronic or mechanical, including photocopying, recording, or by any information storage and retrieval system, without permission in writing from the publisher.

Library of Congress Cataloging-in-Publication Data

Rigal, Natalie.
  [Naissance du goût. English]
  Winning the food fight : how to introduce variety into your child's diet / Natalie Rigal ; translated by Jody Gladding. — 1st U.S. ed.
      p. cm.
  Includes bibliographical references and index.
  ISBN-13: 978-1-59477-097-5 (alk. paper)
  ISBN-10: 1-59477-097-2 (alk. paper)
  1. Children—Nutrition—Psychological aspects. 2. Food habits—Psychological aspects. 3. Food preferences in children. I. Title.
  RJ206.R634 2006
  618.92'39—dc22
                                          2006021689

Printed and bound in the United States by Lake Book Manufacturing

10 9 8 7 6 5 4 3 2 1

Text design and layout by Priscilla Baker and Rachel Goldenberg
This book was typeset in Sabon, with Arepo and Agenda used as display typefaces

31143007782411
618.9239 Rigal
Rigal, Natalie.
Winning the food fight :
how to introduce variety
into your child's diet
1st U.S. ed.

r assistance given by the gov-
of the Ministère de la Culture

; au gouvernement de la France
vre, pour leur concours dans la

Statistical tools can seem like an extension
of the sense organs, allowing us to feel reality.
JEAN-LOUIS R.,
LA VÉRITÉ EST-ELLE SCIENTIFIQUE?
[IS TRUTH SCIENTIFIC?]

I am your extension: the statistics yours, the senses mine. . . .

To Matty Chiva, my professor, for his scientific neophilia.

And also to Achille, Amelle, Armand, Capucine, Charlotte, Claire, Claudia, Clémence, Clément, Clémentine, Domino, Elise, Estelle, Eva, Fanny, François, Héloïse, Inès, Jessica, Jules, Julia, Juliette, Laïla, Lison, Lola, Lucie, Lucien, Marceau, Margaux, Marion, Marouissia, Millie, Mina, Natacha, Nathan, Nicolas, Noé, Paul, Paula, Pauline, Rami, Raphaël (deceased), Sacha, Saëlle, Sam, Sébastien, Solal, Timothé, Ugo, Valentin, Valère, Victor, Anouk (PCC), Louna (BLL), and Yannick (HMV).

I thank Jean-Christophe Brochier for his talent for providing the right sauce for my sometimes astringent remarks.

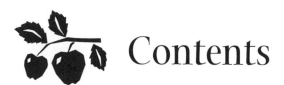

Contents

Introduction

Winning the Food Fight is not the work of a dietitian. I will not discuss calories or a balanced diet or anything like trace elements (a notion that sometimes escapes me). Nor am I a pediatrician. The advice I offer is not a wise, intuitive interpretation of my daily experiences with children and parents. And I have never worked as a psychotherapist of taste. Each individual story is not examined in the light of familial relationships.

I do not refute or criticize any of these approaches to food-related behaviors and difficulties in children. Nevertheless, the one that I propose is different. This book represents the synthesis of my work as a research psychologist specializing in children's taste. Taking a scientific approach, I wanted to answer a simple question: how would one teach children in general, and my daughters in particular, to like vegetables? (I did not write "cauliflower" here because, for reasons I will explain, my daughters are wild about cauliflower.) Of course, this question gave rise to others: Are all children, like mine, often selective in their food choices? Why doesn't this selectivity exist before the age of two?

1

Why are vegetables the prime target of rejection? Why does my eldest daughter detest peas, while my youngest adores them? And on and on . . .

My initial research at university libraries provided this reassuring information: yes, my daughters are normal! Like 77 percent of children between the ages of two and ten, they prove to be selective and conservative in the area of food, rejecting new foods and strictly favoring others (I am speaking especially of a fetish for pasta, of course). Translated into research jargon, this means that food selectivity corresponds to a normal period of child development (in the statistical sense, which does not make the whole business any less difficult).

Perhaps you are saying to yourself, "The conclusion's obvious. It's a necessary stage. Hence, children must be allowed to make their own choices until they understand for themselves that eating too much candy will make them sick. Here's one more psychologist belaboring the idea of respect for children and their differences as the only way to guarantee their autonomy." Well, in fact, no. Developmental psychologists no longer need to defend the child's right to respect; this idea is now widely accepted. Now, children must be spared the torments of too much freedom.

In the area of food especially, the idea of a normal developmental period during which children appear particularly selective must not lead to total permissiveness, resulting in children eating only the dishes they like. There are three good reasons for this: humans are, by nature, omnivorous and need to diversify their diets; to grow is to learn; and eating is a pleasure that we cultivate so that it can cultivate us into social and cultural beings.

Therein lies the paradox. To eat well, one must eat with pleasure, yet children experience only disgust when facing a plate of vegetables. The only way out is to teach them the pleasure of tastes. And not with the help of a course or even of discourse, but as a daily practice, implicitly. And contrary to popular belief, some researchers (myself among them) *are* interested in the question of pleasure, especially in the area of food. The results of their work, analyzed, organized, and synthesized, constitute the heart of this volume. The applications that follow from their fundamental research can be used in everyday life, with our own children.

Quite obviously, there is no magic formula (or recipe, except to add a little cream to the soup sometimes, or not to leave too many strings in the green beans). Yet we do know how certain methods affect the way preferences are established. My goal is to explain them to you so you can teach your children the pleasure of tastes. Be aware, however, that this is no simple matter. There is the average (five-year-olds, for example) and then there are individual differences (your five-year-old). There is no general program that can be applied, good for everyone and for all foods, no matter the circumstances. And in this area as well, education is synonymous with adaptation.

One final word: This book was originally published in France under the title *The Birth of Taste* (La naissance du goût). Indeed, producing this work was a matter of an actual birth, with a long gestation and difficult labor. To understand how food tastes are established among children, many specialties must be broached. I had to force my way into neurophysiology, sensory analysis, and various branches of psychology, sociology, and philosophy. Through the wayward course of my readings, I discovered that there is no real discrepancy between these various specialties,

3

whether they deal with molecules or education. Taste is a sensation that one can learn to experience differently. Even if it may initially seem circuitous, I invite you to follow the route I myself traveled; "to taste" means "to know," and cultivating taste requires many kinds of knowledge.

Bon appétit to the reader on this long gustatory journey.

1

Taste in All the Senses

Look at a dish, then savor it, and your five senses will be awakened by it. Sight tells us about the appearance of the food, its form and color. Taste is used to appreciate its flavors. Smell informs us about its odors, which are released to the nose or circulated in the mouth. Touch evokes the texture of the food, which both the hand and the mouth can sense. Finally, hearing adds a touch of sound to the tactile perception. This already complex scene hides an even greater diversity of stimuli if we consider the trigeminal sensations, which the senses do not register but which we must not fail to mention (and which we will discuss later in this chapter). Thus, food seems to be the most stimulating object for our senses, all contributing to the discovery of its various qualities.

Each of these sensory modes always operates according to three dimensions: quality, intensity, and pleasure. For example, to speak of the odor of a cheese, we would say that its quality is that of a

Muenster or that it "calls up the farm." Its intensity can become more pronounced according to the product's degree of maturity. An older Muenster will emit a stronger odor than its younger version. Finally, the dimension of pleasure involves a judgment—"I like" or "I don't like" the odor of this cheese—which becomes approval: "I will taste" or "I won't taste" this cheese.

Each sensation can thus be traced according to these three dimensions, and they should be kept in mind when you observe your child. Considering all three in relation to one another will help you understand, or even predict, your child's likes and dislikes. The "sweet tooths" and the "thrill seekers" will not choose the same products. The first will prefer Golden Delicious apples, while the second will be particularly drawn to Granny Smiths and tart, juicy russets. If we want to open the path of fruit to them, why not first offer them "their apple," the one that they will enjoy biting into because it delights their taste buds?

To become aware of this sensory multiplicity and to talk about it is also to offer your children the opportunity to enter a secret world overflowing with riches concealed by the banality of the act of eating. I am proposing that you take a few steps, perhaps your first, into the domain of sensorial eating to discover just how stimulating this universe can be.

Look, Touch, Listen

Look: When the Food Appears

Begin by observing the dishes presented to you. When we approach food, sight is the first sense we call upon prior to tasting it. Sight assesses its appearance, that is, its state (solid or liquid), color, and form. Very early on, children learn to identify elementary forms (circles, squares, and triangles) and primary colors (blue, yellow, and red). From these basic categories they will be able to develop a much-larger visual palette. Thanks to this knowledge, children prove perfectly capable of talking about the color and form of a food.

Nevertheless, it is not this type of descriptive attitude that they spontaneously adopt. It is an inquisitive approach that comes to the fore: Is this product "good to eat"? Is it "for me"? Questioning results in a decision: "No, I won't eat this meat, it's too red; this chocolate, it's too dark; this apple, it's too green." These examples show that visual information can tell us about the taste of a food. It tells us how well-done the meat is, how bitter the chocolate, or how sour the fruit.

Such signs are not always reliable, however. The color of a soup does not allow us to predict its exact taste; a biscuit, inadvertently cut in two, is not half as good than in its original state; the few stems of parsley garnishing the dish of green beans do not make them even more unpleasant to eat.

It is nevertheless on the basis of visual examination that children decide whether or not to taste a food presented to them. And parents know that reversing that decision will be no small matter. Thus children must be given the means to find other signs that will sometimes prove more reliable and so better prepare them for the taste of the food. Texture is one of those signs because its qualities are perceptible first by the hand and then in the mouth.

Touch: When the Food Is Fingered and Chewed

Now, touch the food and you will obtain information about its texture. This is first a matter not of the texture in the mouth but of what the hand can feel, either through gentle contact or by applying pressure. Through contact, we caress a piece of fruit and notice the softness of its skin, or we smooth out bread dough and make it presentable. Through pressure, we gauge the ripeness of fruit or cheese or the crispness of a baguette, and thus how well-baked it is.

In the mouth, texture unfolds as well. It is no longer a matter of what the hand perceives in caressing or fingering the product but a matter of the texture perceived by the oral cavity. Simple contact with the food tells us something about its most prominent tactile modes, like stickiness. As for chewing, it allows us to differentiate the various nuances on a basic scale going from soft to hard: crumbly, flaky, chewy, crispy, crunchy, and many more.

Texture becomes an important topic when the first bits of meat are introduced into the daily diets of infants six months to two years old. Ergonomic questions concerning teeth and swallowing capacity most certainly play a part in the relationship between young children and the texture of their foods.

But beyond this ergonomic approach, texture often remains a neglected mode in our assessment of foods. Through studies done with children, however, it appears that texture helps predict their preferences. The difference in texture helps explain why 49 percent of children like cauliflower when it is prepared in a béchamel sauce, as opposed to only 35 percent when it is offered in a salad. In the latter case, however, a new sense also contributes: the ear reacts to the crunchiness of raw cauliflower.

Listen: When the Food Is Heard

Now close your eyes and listen. A new sensorial dimension comes into play: hearing. As with touch, hearing informs us about food both before it enters and once it is inside the mouth. Heard externally, certain foods make noise: boiling soup, bubbles bursting in champagne, a bread crust giving way under the pressure of a hand. Heard internally, noises contribute to the perception of texture: chewing reveals the crispness of an apple or the elasticity of chewing gum.

Hearing remains the least essential sense in the discovery of the sensory richness of food, all the more so because we live in an age in which noises emitted from the mouth are discouraged ("Eat with your mouth shut!"). During a recent cultural event ("the Taste of Darkness"), audience volunteers sampled a menu in a room that was totally dark. The accounts of their experience, gathered at the end of the meal, attest to the importance given to auditory stimulation in recognizing foodstuffs. Rendered blind, these tasters also testified to paying very particular attention to the odor of the foods before ingesting them.

Smelling the Odors

Bring a dish to your nose and breathe in: the world of smells is offered to you. This is a sensory world of infinite richness because each dish releases a specific scent, varying in complexity. Now take the dish into your mouth and relocate the odors that you have just breathed in. Just like tactile and auditory perceptions, olfactory sensations can arise not only before but also during the tasting.

Those Odors We Breathe In

This is an everyday act, if less and less common: bringing an object to one's nose and taking a whiff. Through this act, our sense of smell investigates the odor of the food (sometimes called the "scent" when it is perceived through the nose). When we breathe in, an air current passes through the nasal cavity, conveying volatile odiferous molecules. Coming into contact with a receptor organ located in the nose, the nasal epithelium, these molecules produce an olfactory sensation.

The objective of this act can be twofold. First, it can be a way of protecting oneself from ingesting products that might have gone bad, as when one sniffs milk to check whether it has curdled, or from ingesting inedible products, as when the irritating sensations of ammonia released from a bottle make one hold it away. Thus, smelling a product often contributes to an attitude of mistrust.

But this gesture can encompass an entirely different attitude, one that seeks out pleasure. There again, as we approach the product without ingesting it, by trying to identify it, by comparing it to something familiar, by recalling pleasant memories, our appetite is, in the end, stimulated.

All such behavior preceding ingestion permits us to formulate hypotheses regarding the food's taste, that is, what we risk experiencing by taking the food in. This behavior can also be observed at the market, where certain shoppers turn products over, examine them, and sniff them in order to choose the best possible foods. Proceeding in this manner, they sometimes make good hypotheses. But that is not always the case. From time to time, there is some discrepancy between the product's smell when it is held in one's hand and the odor it releases in one's mouth.

Those Odors We Taste

Contrary to general belief, odor is not perceived only before tasting; it is also perceived once the food enters the mouth. The eater is capable of perceiving odors thanks to a passage linking the back of the throat to the nasal cavity. At that point, we can no longer speak of the odor detected by the nose, known as the scent, but of the odor detected in the mouth, sometimes called the aroma.

Scents and aromas develop according to similar patterns. In both cases, the scented molecules of the food come in contact with the receptor cells of the nasal epithelium. This parallel pattern leads to a perceptive continuity between scents and aromas. Thus, in general, smelling a piece of ripe fruit and tasting it produce nearly identical olfactory sensations. But in some cases chewing (and thus breaking down), warming, or cooling a food can change that perception significantly.

There are many examples illustrating the discrepancy between odors for the mouth and odors for the nose. Strawberries bought at market can have a very delicate scent that somehow seems to fade when they are tasted. Certain cheeses like Muenster offer a very strong odor to the nose and another, much less intense one in the mouth. Alternately, certain wines develop a more powerful bouquet when they are tasted than when they are simply sniffed. Temperature actually alters the proportion of an odor's constituents and thus our ultimate perception of it. The other constituent element in taste, that is, flavor, also varies in quality according to the temperature of the food.

Tasting the Flavors

Now, take the time to savor this exquisite dish and appreciate its flavors. Learn how to make the most of these rare moments because only foods can lead you along the gustatory way.

The Four Flavors and Beyond

After odor, the second sensation experienced in the mouth is flavor. It is produced by what are called sapid molecules that are perceived by receptors located on the tongue, also known as taste buds. There are four types of taste buds, and that is one reason why it was long thought that only four taste sensations existed.

Indeed, eaters like ourselves are in the habit of dividing tastes into four well-known categories: sweet, salty, sour, and bitter. This habit dates back to at least the beginning of the twentieth century, when physiologist Hans Henning began to describe gustatory sensations. This researcher effectively demonstrated that these four terms were indispensable for describing the sensation of taste. But most important, he demonstrated that each gustatory sensation can be represented within a geometric form composed of four vertices, corresponding to sweet, salty, sour, and bitter. Thus, it is an extreme simplification to confine our taste sensations to these four notions individually when, in reality, flavor is most often located at the intersection of several of them. Even aspartame, that sugar substitute you drop into your coffee, is both sweet and bitter. Today's researchers, Annick Faurion among them, offer experimental data that confirms the truly continuous nature of gustatory sensation.

These researchers reveal to us an even more complex reality regarding our taste sensations. Numerous flavors exist for which we simply do not have names. Take licorice, for example. Licorice has little odor; it is mostly the tongue that it stimulates. People tend to describe its taste as "sweet," to the extent that they associate it with the realm of confectioner's products. But no objective descriptor exists for naming the flavor released by licorice.

Even though they do not always refer to a tangible biological reality, the four descriptors—sweet, salty, sour, and bitter—are found in a multitude of languages. Only a few exceptional cultures introduce other sapid descriptors, notably the Japanese. The Japanese language has at its disposal a fifth taste, umami, which refers to the specific flavor of glutamate, sometimes described in the East as a gustatory sensation between sweet, salty, and sour; for the Japanese, it constitutes a taste all to itself.

It is nevertheless true that these four canonical terms remain firmly entrenched in our everyday vocabulary, and each of them evokes references more or less precise and individual. For sweet, the reference for everyone is sucrose, a product available in all stores and which we use primarily in the preparation of desserts. For salty, of course, the reference is salt, which is added to our dishes to enhance their flavor. Sour does not correspond to any easily identifiable manufactured product. The perception of sourness derives from the activation of taste buds by the ion $H+$. But in our everyday psychology, references are vague, even if most of us are tempted to mention lemons or vinegar as prototypical acidic products. There is also the tendency to find products as diverse as mustard and champagne acidic because of a long-established semantic confusion between "sharp" and "sour." We will see, however, that pungent sensations are not taste sensations.

As for bitter, things become even more confusing here, because even for scientists no single precise reference exists. We don't know what bitter is, unless it is a solution of quinine, something we practically never mix into food. No foodstuffs contain it. Nevertheless, the term "bitter" is commonly used to describe the taste of dark chocolate, and also beer, endive, and coffee. But the molecular structures of those four products are not comparable. In reality, the term "bitter," supposedly a sensory descriptor in our language, plays the role of a hedonic descriptor, especially for children. It describes not a sensation but, in this case, a displeasure. In other words, children will tend to describe as "bitter" products they do not like.

Finally, with regard to the terms "acid" and "bitter," adults often confuse intensity and quality. For a product that offers a very pronounced taste, they tend to use these terms interchangeably, even when that product evokes neither acidity nor, for something like coffee, bitterness.

In summary, in everyday psychology, the terms "sweet" and "salty" are generally used appropriately to describe products to which sugar or salt has been added. On the other hand, "sour" and "bitter" form the basis for many confusions, especially between quality, intensity, and pleasure. The term "taste" itself is the subject of much confusion.

Taste for Eaters and Taste for Scientists

The term "taste" is used differently according to whether one is talking among friends or one is presenting a paper at a scientific conference. For scientists, taste is a sensory modality that can be broken down into specific flavors. That is how we have just been discussing it. But for eaters, the term encompasses all the sensations perceived in the mouth, including flavors, odors, and even textures, which in combination produce a unique sensation that determines our assessment ("I like [or I don't like] the taste of this food").

To speak of the blend of taste and smell, and to avoid the inconveniences of the multiple meanings of the word "taste," scientists use the term "flavor." This word is very accommodating. It allows for objectivity to play some part in subjective psychology to the extent that the sensory convergence between flavors and odors is so great that it is impossible to perceive them separately from one another. This explains the difficulty we face in assigning roles to taste in its strict sense—sweet, salty, sour, and bitter—and smell.

Thus, when you bite into a raspberry fruit drop, you experience a unique sensation, a result of the combination of the artificial raspberry and the extreme sweetness. You do not experience the raspberry aroma as one thing and the taste of sweetness as another.

In reality, at least for the tastes of sweet and salty, flavors are very rarely experienced alone. They are always accompanied by more or less powerful smells. As evidence, consider how a simple cold, that is, congestion in the nasal cavity, leads to the loss of smell and is enough to make us lose our bearings with regard to food sensations. We say that food has no taste (we should say "no smell"). In fact, we can no longer perceive odor in the mouth, which represents about 80 percent of the information of a taste (and some products, like cumin and vanilla, are all smell). To return to the fruit drop example, in the case of a cold, whether it is artificial raspberry, lemon, or even mint, the candy will "taste" the same to you, because you will be aware only of its sweet nature. On the other hand, if by accident you became agueusic, that is, you lost the ability to taste, a bitter orange and a sweet orange would produce the same sensations.

From now on we will be vigilant about distinguishing between the two types of taste, so as not to confuse these two processes. "Taste" will refer to taste as it breaks down into sweet, salty, sour, and bitter, and "flavor" will refer to taste as that whole ensemble of gustatory and olfactory sensations that produce a unique sensation. But before discussing a third sense of the term (taste-pleasure), we must mention the existence of a sixth sense that collaborates internally with smell and taste to produce our perceptions of flavor.

A Sixth Sense

Other sensory modes, of which we are even less in the habit of speaking, also play a part in how a product tastes. And the most important of these, which we can call a true sixth sense, is responsible for the perception of chemical sensations known as trigeminals.

The name is certainly barbaric, but our current language has no other way of designating this sense. It owes its origin to the nerve that conveys trigeminal information, that is, the trigeminal nerve. This nerve is located at the back of the throat, close to the olfactory bulb. This location gives it the ability to react to both nasal (smelled by the nose) and oral (tasted by the mouth) stimuli.

The trigeminal nerve turns out to be responsible for the irritating, even painful sensations produced by condiments and spices like black pepper, red pepper, curry, ginger, and mustard. It reacts to the carbonation in soft drinks as well as to alcohol. It also responds, by revolting, to the irritating sensation of ammonia. Finally, it conveys to the brain the sensory impressions of nicotine, as well as the painful impressions produced by a toothache.

Clearly, this unrecognized sense collaborates in our everyday perceptions. It keeps us informed in the kitchen when we prepare a dressing, throughout the day when we smoke to satisfy a craving, and in the laundry when we use certain household products. It provides sensations as diverse as spicy, pungent, metallic, burning, biting, stinging, and fizzy. This is a matter not of taste or smell but of absolutely specific sensations that make us say, generally, that the product is "sharp" or "has a bite." But the bite of mustard and that of very cold sparkling water are two different sensations; one would have to be described as burning and the other as fizzy.

All these impressions are sometimes designated by the expression "That's strong." The reason for this may be that elevated gustatory or olfactory concentrations become irritating. It appears that most chemical compounds can stimulate the trigeminal nerve if they are introduced in high enough concentrations.

Still other sensations exist as well, most notably thermal ones, which routinely play a role because they alter our perception of smells and tastes. Depending on temperature, a product may be perceived as more or less sweet because the intensity of sweetness is heightened when a food is hot. Thus some of us prefer our apple pie cold because it is easier to bite right into a cold pie and it rarely seems too sweet.

We appear to have reached the end of our wanderings in the land of taste. I hope this tour has filled you with all the sensory impressions that can be experienced, for example, by tasting a cream-filled pastry: the shape at once elongated and plump; its chestnut color, more or less dark; its crust smooth and soft to the touch; in the mouth, the taste very sweet, the flavor hinting of chocolate or coffee, its texture creamy and a little sticky. It seems that taste is a veritable sensory bouquet of infinite richness. Yet humans, trained to use their eyes to decipher the world around them, will still sometimes choose their foods according to appearance rather than taste.

Between Appearance and Taste

Food is consumed first of all by the eyes. And that is sometimes a mistake, because while taste is the very essence of food, humans often grant sight a dominant role in making their judgments. Food sensations come into play, of course, at two times: before food enters the mouth, with shape, color, touch, and smell; and during the tasting, through the subtle mix of tastes and smells supplemented by tactile and trigeminal impressions. It is true that visual impressions precede taste impressions in the chronology of the eating act. Nevertheless, appearance does not always lead to good predictions about the flavor of food.

Appearances Are Sometimes Deceiving

The color of a food is almost always the first characteristic to be evaluated. However, it is not necessarily a very reliable indicator of the flavor. For example, we choose strawberries according to their color, looking for the reddest ones possible. But the reddest strawberries are not always the tastiest or the most flavorful in the mouth. Similarly, we choose certain products according to their aesthetic appearance. But a beautiful bright green avocado, with its shiny skin, will not necessarily be the best of the lot. On the contrary, sometimes rusty brown indicates good-quality flavor.

The first sensations we experience when encountering a certain food may prove to be deceiving. Some people have known this for a long time and have tried to profit by it. To stay with our example of strawberries, it is clear that their color and their more or less beautiful appearance are not always good indicators of the taste they will produce in the mouth. But strawberry producers know how consumers choose their products—that is, solely according to visual appearances and without tasting them. So they try to create new species, as rich in color as possible and with the most attractive forms. In market stands, sellers use special lighting designed to make their fruit shine. But in our own kitchens, without the help of these ploys, products often lose their appeal.

And what is true for the behavior of adults is even more true for children. Marketing teams and those who work in the research and development sectors for children's products are very much aware of this. They are particularly attentive to the appearance of their products, which, in large part, determines children's decisions. Looking at food, even unfamiliar food, children voice hypotheses regarding the taste and are capable of deciding whether or not they will like it. If a child decides she won't like a food, it will be very difficult just to make her agree to taste it. And if she agrees to that, her parents will have the hardest time altering her anticipated judgment. Even when she does not find the food so bad after all, she may well decide that it is not for her. It will be necessary to repeat the experience a certain number of times to bring her around to revising her initial judgment.

Many studies conducted on the link between judgments made visually and in the mouth show that adults and children can be easily deceived. For example, in 1994 Marie-Odile Monneuse studied the impact of the color of fruit pastries on the hedonic judgment of adults and children. In other words, with all the products offered having the same flavor (apple and the identical concentration of sugar), were the fruit pastries more or less favored according to their color?

For the majority of the subjects questioned, the pastries most preferred were the red ones. For example, those were the ones that children spontaneously chose when they were allowed to select among five options. Moreover, the red and purple pastries were judged to be sweeter than the yellow and green ones. What to conclude? Certainly that the children had had some previous experiences whereby they had learned to associate the color red with sweet fruit and the color green with less ripe, and thus less sweet, fruit.

Another type of experiment was conducted by Frédéric Brochet with enologists in their last year of training. These specialists were taught to use completely different terms to evoke the sensory qualities of wines of different colors. In other words, the lexical palette for red wines is not the same as that for white wines. Brochet colored various white wines red and asked the winemakers to describe their sensations as they normally would. Most of them were fooled and used the terms reserved for red wines.

Similarly, Brochet presented them with some fine vintage wines in the plastic bottles used for mediocre wines. Once again, the winemakers were deceived and pronounced mostly negative judgments. Conversely, when he poured a rough red wine into a bottle bearing the label of a very good wine, the enologists generally described it as excellent.

These two experiments offer good evidence that our sensory perceptions are subjective, and that previous experience can play a determining role, even for specialists whose job it is to analyze the sensory qualities of products. They show how we create hypotheses about what we are going to taste and the importance of these hypotheses, especially for children, who subsequently have the most difficulty adjusting their perceptions to the actual taste they perceive. Very often, they perceive it as they thought it should be.

The Taste of Darkness, that artistic event we have already mentioned, shows the extent to which vision conditions our food perceptions. Through the unusual situation of dining in the company of a blind person and other guests in absolute darkness, the normal interplay of the senses is jumbled. Without the aid of the eye, the perception of taste becomes murky; reference points must be reinvented. It is by attempting to recognize foods under these conditions that one becomes fully conscious of sounds, smells, and flavors.

In normal situations, children trust the appearance of food when making judgments about its taste. They must be given the means to understand that "beautiful" does not mean "good." In this regard, sensory education should offer them a way to approach food from a new angle. We have already mentioned the principles of sensory education and will later present the basic formulas for it. Children who become attentive to odors, for example, will no longer choose foods solely by their color, an indicator that is sometimes deceptive. Thus, they will be able to savor fully in their mouths the taste of the food.

Taste: A Hedonic Judgment

The word "taste" in our language assumes quite a complex assortment of multiple meanings, resulting in many misunderstandings. We have already discussed the confusion between taste and flavor. And staying within the sensory domain, we have just seen how taste in the mouth is often associated with the taste of the eye. The whole array of visual, tactile, gustatory, olfactory, trigeminal, and auditory impressions tends to be harmonized into a unique sensory image.

But beyond the purely sensory sphere, taste always finds itself implicated in an aesthetic judgment or, more precisely, what is called a hedonic judgment—that is to say, one that refers to the dimension of pleasure and thus to the fact that something is either liked or disliked. In other words, any discussion about a food's taste leads us very quickly to considerations regarding the plea-sure we experience (or do not) in eating it. From a taste *of* the food on a sensory level, we move to a taste *for* the food, a hedonic judgment.

How does this transition from taste-sense to taste-pleasure take place? To answer that question, we must understand what pleasure is from a physiological perspective. Today, that is more or less pos-sible. Professor Patrick MacLeod explains the pleasure center as a network of subcortical cells that exhibit the peculiarity of both being nonspecific and serving as integrators. They are nonspecific because they receive very diverse information: sensory in nature (received from each of the six senses); originating from the vis-cera (which inform the person about the effects of food on the body); and also originating from the conditions under which food is consumed (physical, social, and emotional). They are integrators because, within this network of cells, a unique sensory impression is formed, resulting from the combined input of the six senses, plus the perceived effects on the body and the context of consumption.

A hedonic value is assigned to the condensed image of the tasted food, that is, a mark of pleasure or displeasure. These two bits of data are stored together in the memory. When a person again confronts the food, he will do some mnemonic research, looking for the condensed impression. Inevitably, the hedonic value with which it has been associated will surface at the same time. If this stored value is positive, he will engage in pursuit behavior and consume the food. In the opposite case, if the hedonic value turns out to be negative, he will avoid consuming it.

We now understand better the shift from taste-sense to taste-pleasure. In a single process, the human organism registers the con-densed sensory impression and the pleasure. When that memory is reactivated, we can simply examine a food and know whether or not we are willing to eat it. Thus, the sensory impressions the chocolate cream puff gives rise to—the fact that it is nourishing or that it once made you sick, the friendly or unfriendly atmosphere of the bakery you frequent, and the pastry's suggestion of a world of round creaminess (a world you embrace or reject)—can render it more or less appealing to you. This is a measure of the great complexity of the alimentary act, which is governed by a kind of pleasure that encompasses simultaneously sensory aspects, nutritive aspects, and the context of consumption.

The origin of the shift from "taste of" (sensory) to "taste for" (hedonic) also may be rooted in the fact that taste is the single sensory mode that includes a genetic inscription for pleasure. That is to say, it is linked with a primary emotional response. From the first days of life, certain tastes universally give pleasure, while others are rejected from birth, both here and elsewhere.

2
Taste and the Genes

I s taste innate? In other words, is there a genetic program inscribed in the human organism that leads humans to exhibit certain aversions or preferences for foods? The question is posed on two levels: the general level of the species and the specific level of the individual and family heredity.

Actually, our genetic inheritance is located at each of these levels: the level of the human species, which determines that each human has eyes to see with, and the level of the particular individual, resulting from the encounter of the mother's and father's genes, which determines that certain individuals will have blue eyes and others brown eyes. Thus a universal and an individual and familial heredity are combined in each of us, from which we must deduce the effects upon food tastes.

Genes and the Omnivore

In the first stage of our inquiry, we must ask whether the omnivore is equipped to accept or reject certain food substances according to their sensory characteristics. We will investigate first tastes and then smells, examining whether some of them are subject to universal acceptance or rejection.

The Omnivore in the Land of Tastes

A group of studies focuses on the reactions of infants introduced to the four canonical tastes (sweet, salty, sour, and bitter). The studies generally consist of making newborns taste sapid molecules diluted in water—sucrose, salt, citric acid, and quinine successively—and then observing their reactions. The reactions of very young infants are manifested in various ways. Sometimes there are behavioral indications, like ingestion or the orientation of the head. Sometimes there are physiological changes, variations in heart rate and breathing, for example.

These studies establish that infants' reactions are clearly differentiated according to whether the taste is sweet, salty, sour, or bitter, which means that they know how to recognize these different tastes, even without being able to name them.

Some researchers, Matty Chiva in France among them, are interested in one particularly strong indication, called the gusto-facial reflex. This is a reflex, universal and unconditioned, that is manifested from birth by typical facial expressions, expressions identical among all individuals but different according to the sapid solutions introduced.

What do these expressions look like? For sucrose solutions, the face is relaxed, almost smiling; the baby displays sucking motions, with the tip of the tongue sometimes protruding toward the upper lip. A very different expression appears for solutions of citric acid, characterized by pursing and protruding the lips, squinting the eyes, and wrinkling the nose. For bitter solutions of quinine sulfate, the mouth is open, the upper lip is arched, the tongue is very visible and flat, and the baby salivates; sometimes there are movements similar to those that precede vomiting. Finally, with a salt solution, the baby's expression depends upon the concentration of the salt; a very weak solution will prompt an undifferentiated expression that is difficult to interpret; with a very strong solution, the expression resembles that manifested by infants tasting an acid solution.

If you take photos of infants in the process of reacting to these different sapid solutions and you ask uninformed individuals what the infants are feeling at the moment of the snapshot, they will almost unanimously tell you that the child is experiencing pleasure for the sweet solution and displeasure for the sour, bitter, and strong salt solutions.

The gusto-facial reflex thus permits us to recognize that infants universally tend to accept the sweet taste and to reject the sour, bitter, and too salty tastes. This reflex is the obvious manifestation of a genetic inscription for pleasure and displeasure in response to certain tastes. The early appearance of the gusto-facial reflex (from the first days of life) and its universal nature (all infants everywhere react in the same way) indicate that it really is an unconditioned phenomenon, unrelated to any learning.

Moreover, most researchers recognize an adaptive function in this inscription. They now hold that the genetic inscription for sweetness allows the infant to be better fed during the first months of life, since mother's milk, as we all know, is slightly sweet. Similarly, they think that the rejection of bitterness provides protection against poisoning by many toxic products that possess this disagreeable taste.

No Genetic Inscription for Odors

Young human beings possess very sensitive olfactory capabilities. From the first hours of life, they are able to recognize their mother's bodily scent. If they are breastfed, they will know how to tell the difference between the odor of their own mother's milk and the milk of some other mother. Is this precocious ability to discriminate linked to preestablished hedonic reactions inscribed in the genome?

As with tastes, it was long thought that a genetic inscription existed for pleasure and displeasure with regard to smells. It is true that in a given culture children and adults classify good and bad smells according to an almost identical pattern. For example, children and adults in the West are in general agreement about rejecting the smell of excrement and appreciating the smell of vanilla. However, that consensus is far from established until the age of three or sometimes even the age of five, according to certain studies. Before that age, there are individual examples of appreciation apparent through basic observation. Thus, some babies might accept the odor of vanilla and reject that of excrement, as opposed to other babies who will turn their heads away from vanilla and not modify their behavior at the smell of excrement.

One French researcher, Benoist Schaal, proposed a hypothesis according to which the differences among individual olfactory preferences at birth are partly the consequence of intrauterine experiences. Schaal's idea is that during gestation the baby ingests amniotic fluid and thus gradually becomes familiar with certain odors linked to the foods the mother consumes. At birth, apparently, the newborn cannot distinguish the odor of the mother's amniotic fluid from that of her colostrum (also bearing the odors of ingested foods). Thus, olfactory preferences acquired during gestation would prepare the fetus for its new food diet, that is, the mother's milk.

Such preferences would be "innate" in the strict sense of the term ("what can be observed at birth") but not in its wider sense ("inscribed in the genetic inheritance"). Moreover, most researchers now share the idea that there are no genetically determined good or bad odors. In fact, the rejection of bad odors is quite closely related to experience, much more so, in any case, than the rejection of acidity or bitterness—at least insofar as observation has shown.

Let us note nevertheless that the innate inscription for a hedonic response to tastes, as interesting as it is, actually provides very little information, as it involves only four tastes and is expressed only in absolute terms: I like, I do not like. The learning experiences that infants go through allow for these initial reactions to diversify and for certain meanings to be assigned to the sapid messages. Even if children are universally programmed to reject acidity, they can very well come to appreciate this taste as they gain experience.

Finally, in matters of food behavior, learning experiences remain paramount. First, in the light of current knowledge, the hedonic response to odors does not appear to be genetically determined. Second, the four basic tastes certainly produce specific, unconditioned, and universal responses, but those responses evolve over the course of ongoing daily experiences with food. For the human species, this flexibility may have an adaptive function. As omnivores, humans are born with very few innate preferences and aversions. They are led to choose what suits them from nutritional and hedonic perspectives, and this allows them at the same time to adapt to their environments. Moreover, each individual makes these choices within a given cultural environment. These individual characteristics may be evidence of a genetic inheritance specific to each one of us.

Genes and the Individual

This is a question asked regularly in numerous contexts: does genetics explain the attitudes and behaviors that parents and children share? To answer this question in the context of sports, for example, we must first examine whether the members of a family actually practice the same sports activities. If that proves true, we can then go on to try to explain similarities according to transmittable physical aptitudes, like agility, strength, or stamina.

In the area of food, we can proceed in the same fashion by first examining the degree of resemblance between the parents' and children's tastes. Then we can look for genetic characteristics that could explain a possible commonality of tastes within the family.

Preferences and Aversions: The Paradox of the Family

At one time or another, each of us has wondered whether tastes and distastes are inherited from our parents in the same way that eye color is. It is a difficult issue to resolve, all the more so because it can be approached through so many different methods. One can, for example, focus on a single generation and undertake what are called gemellary studies. This is a matter of observing the preferences and aversions of twins, and asking whether the preferences of identical twins more closely resemble one another than the preferences of fraternal twins, or even of brothers and sisters who are not twins.

Four major studies have attempted to answer this question, producing very contradictory results. The first revolved around solutions of sucrose (sweet taste) and sodium chloride (salty taste) dissolved in water. It showed that the preferences of 146 pairs of identical twins did not resemble each other any more than the preferences of 165 pairs of fraternal twins, which would indicate that genetic inheritance does not strictly dictate the preferences of young children for sapid solutions.

Three other studies focused on actual foods and not on sapid solutions. The first showed that the hedonic responses to twenty-three different foods were not more varied for thirty-four pairs of fraternal twins than for thirty-eight pairs of identical twins, except in the case of foods that produced spicy trigeminal sensations. On the contrary, the second study, focusing on 101 different foods, revealed clearer preferences between identical twins than between fraternal twins. Finally, the last study demonstrated that some preferences might be inherited, depending upon the foods. For just a third of the foods (eight out of twenty-four) in this last study, the tastes of identical twins were more similar than the tastes of fraternal twins.

Another way to study family heredity, this time crossing generations, is to focus on the preferences and aversions that children and parents share. Centering on young children, a study conducted in 1980 established that, for all kinds of foods, only 10 percent of the correlations between the preferences of children and of their mothers are significant. That figure drops to 6 percent for significant correlations between the preferences of children and their fathers. On the other hand, a study conducted in 1986 showed that there are stronger correlations between the food preferences of brothers and sisters than there are between the food preferences of children belonging to the same cultural group but to different families.

Other researchers have subsequently focused on older subjects, especially adolescents. In general, the degree of resemblance between the preferences of children and their parents increases with the age of the children. The tastes of adolescents are closer to those of their parents than the tastes of children are. Nevertheless, throughout a dozen American studies, the correlation rate remained weak and never passed the threshold of 50 percent. In some other respects, one American study proved to be particularly interesting. It showed weaker correlations between parents and adolescents with regard to food tastes than with regard to moral values (religion and politics) or aesthetics (cultural, literary, musical, and other preferences). This means that, contrary to popular belief, each of us is actually much more influenced by our parents on the moral and artistic levels than on the level of food.

The various studies conducted on the role of family heredity in food preferences are too few and often incomplete, and they do not always produce corroborating results. Nevertheless, we can at least draw the following conclusions from them: First, correlations among members of the same family fall more on the side of aversions than preferences, and they are even more significant for strong and certain spicy or even bitter sensations, as we will see. Second, the studies all seem to indicate a weak genetic determinism in the establishment of food preferences, thus once more underlining the importance of learning experiences.

This last result is nonetheless surprising. On the one hand, given the close links between diet and biology, we could have expected a much more pronounced genetic determinism. On the other hand, because parents and children eat most of their meals together, that should tend to make them appreciate the same dishes. Correlations between parents' and children's tastes do not follow this pattern, which is why one American psychologist, Paul Rozin, refers to this subject as "the paradox of the family." Few studies offer an explanation of this paradox. The only factor that seems to shed light on it is the degree of similarity between the father's and mother's tastes, known as the degree of parental congruence. This allows us to construct some interesting hypotheses. For example, it may be that when parents have very different tastes from each other, their children do not exhibit a strong family identity in terms of food.

The existence of such a paradox in preferences should lead us to formulate a strong hypothesis on the absence of familial genetic determinism in food tastes. Taste-preference, however, is not taste-sensation, and if we do not like the same foods our parents like, it may be that we do not perceive them the same way on the sensory level.

A Sensory World of One's Own

Our parents may not transmit their food tastes to us directly. Still, it is true that, just as they transmit to us hair or eye color in an undeniably genetic fashion, the two of them together determine our degree of sensory sensitivity.

What is sensory sensitivity? The capacity of our receptors, or our sensory organs, to process the information that comes from all around us. According to their makeup, we are more or less sensitive to odors and tastes. Thus those receptor organs, the tongue and the nose, constituted differently according to the individual, will not react in the same way to the various kinds of molecules.

As a function of these physiological differences, the electrical messages conveyed to the brain will differ according to the individual, giving rise to sensations unique to each of us. Modern technology—especially MRIs (magnetic resonance imaging)—makes visual the images formed by electrical messages in our brains. For taste, strong differences can be noted according to the individual, which is not always true for sight and hearing. We might even imagine that if we were lent someone else's eyes, we would not be surprised by what we saw. On the other hand, lent a nose or a tongue, we would be totally astonished by the sensations we experienced, being very different from what our own tongue and nose usually allowed us to sense. This great variability in the makeup of our receptors applies to quantity, or intensity, and also to sensory quality.

Tastes of Variable Intensity

At the level of gustatory intensity, the threshold for detecting a molecule can vary widely from one individual to the next. Take sucrose and dilute it in water in increasing concentrations (the first glass containing 0.2 grams of sucrose per liter of water, the second 0.4 grams, etc.). Have people taste these different solutions and ask them to note the concentration at which they first perceive the sweet quality of the drink. Some people will perceive it with the first glass (0.2 g/l), while others will become aware of it at 1.4 g/l. Results like these, obtained by French researcher Annick Faurion, indicate that the sensitivity of adults to sucrose varies according to a minimum factor of seven.

The observation of great variability among individuals with

regard to taste sensitivity can be applied in educating the palate. Staying with the example of sweet, if a child is hypersensitive to the taste of sucrose, she may put only half a spoonful of sugar in her cereal. On the other hand, a child who proves less sensitive to sucrose will probably need three spoonfuls of sugar to make his cereal acceptable. This example shows us how certain food behaviors can be illuminated by considering congenital factors. Sensory sensitivity is inscribed in our genetic inheritance and may influence our food tastes, as certain studies done on young children seem to suggest.

For example, in studying the gusto-facial reflex among newborns, Matty Chiva also noted that, aside from the universal responses to the four basic tastes, there were very different reaction thresholds according to the individual. Certain infants, for instance, reacted to very weak concentrations of certain bitter solutions, whereas for others the concentration had to be multiplied ten times to produce a gusto-facial reflex worthy of the name.

Chiva went on to follow thirty-four infants from birth to two years of age. His observations allowed him to conclude that five of them were hypogeusic (having gustatory sensations of weak intensity), twenty-one normal, and eight hypergeusic (having very strong gustatory sensations). A questionnaire addressed to their mothers testified that the five hypogeusic children presented no food problems and ate anything as long as they were hungry. On the other hand, the eight hypergeusic children were described as temperamental during meals and difficult in their food choices. They had very marked preferences, exhibited very selective behavior, and refused to taste new products. The study did not extend beyond two years, but the most difficult children may have become fine gourmets as adults!

Even though this study is not sufficient grounds for a definitive verdict, we can assume there is a link between sensory sensitivity and food preferences. Because the least sensitive people feel sensations much less strongly, they prove to be more open in their food choices. For example, they more easily accept the taste of Muenster cheese, which produces a relatively subtle sensation for them in the mouth, whereas for the most sensitive people the sensation will be more intense.

The whole business becomes more complicated when we consider that a person's sensitivity to sucrose may not be the same as his or her sensitivity to fructose, for instance. The degree of gustatory sensitivity depends on the tastes actually present, which implies that grouping people as hyper- or hypogeusic presents some problems. Finally, to complete this already complex scenario, let us add that not just the intensity but also the quality of tastes can be perceived differently according to the individual.

Tastes of Variable Quality

Sensory intensity is not the only thing that varies from one individual to the next. The quality of the sensation varies as well, also because of the makeup of the receptor organs responsible for the perception of tastes and smells, the tongue and nose respectively. With regard to tastes, we can clearly recognize molecules that prompt consensus: sucrose is universally described as sweet and sodium chloride as salty. On the other hand, the population is divided on other tastes. Offer a significant number of people aspartame to taste, and some will describe the product as sweet, while others, very adamantly, will describe it as bitter. The first group may like diet sodas, while the second group will most certainly reject them. There is no perceptual error in either group.

The molecule is perceived differently by these people according to the makeup of their taste buds.

In the domain of tastes, we must pause to consider an interesting molecule called phenylthiocarbamide (PTC). This molecule divides the population into two groups: the tasters and the nontasters. The tasters (about 75 percent of the European population) perceive an almost bitter and therefore disagreeable taste when they experience PTC. As for the nontasters, they perceive PTC only in very strong concentrations. PTC is present in sulfated products, especially cruciferous vegetables like cabbage. That could explain why a great majority of children do not like cauliflower. It may be a matter of the PTC-tasting 75 percent of the population for whom this food produces a disagreeable sensation: Nontasting children would not have better character than the others but would simply be constituted to accept this product, which prompts no displeasure in them.

PTC tasters also prove to be particularly sensitive to a whole family of bitter-tasting chemical compounds (especially propylthiouracil, or more specifically 6-n-proply-2-thiouracil). They prove more sensitive to caffeine and certain trigeminal sensations like the hotness of red pepper. Finally, certain hypertasters of bitter are also hypertasters of sweet. The multisensitivities of some tasters may explain why they demonstrate a much greater propensity for rejecting foods than nontasters do.

However, all the work done on the link between PTC perception and food preferences among adults does not confirm the idea that tasters prove particularly selective in their choices. Learning may still play a part on this level. Just as many adults come to appreciate sour or spicy-hot products through the course of their experiences with foods, so tasters learn to accept a whole spectrum of tastes they initially rejected. Nevertheless, among children, who are less experienced in the domain of foods, the link between sensory sensitivity and food preferences still appears pronounced. Young PTC tasters have yet to learn to accept its bitter taste.

This example clearly shows that as individuals, we each evolve in our own individual world of taste associated with our own unique genetic inheritance. Like hair or eye color, the ability to perceive PTC is the result of the combination of paternal and maternal genes. Becoming aware of the variability of gustatory perceptions among individuals allows us to understand why one child strongly rejects certain foods that seem completely acceptable to other children.

With regard to smells, there is a phenomenon known as anosmia, now clearly described from the neurosensory perspective. Certain individuals with anosmia are not "equipped" to perceive particular smells. Thus, within the French population, one out of ten individuals cannot perceive the odor produced by musk. For androsterone, things are a bit more complicated. Fifty percent of people describe it as having the odor of pee, while the other 50 percent do not perceive this odor at all, unless it is presented in a concentration seven hundred times stronger than the initial one. These people then describe it as having the smell of mildew. These observations were all reported by Patrick MacLeod in an article titled "Si on ne sent pas pareil, c'est qu'on 'nez' pas pareil" ["If one does not smell the same, it is because one is not 'nosed' the same"]. The pun on the homophones *nez* (nose) and *naît* (is born) very clearly aims at advancing the genetic character of some of our olfactory perceptions.

Thus we might conclude this chapter by reiterating that all humans, as omnivores, are programmed first to choose their foods and adapt to their environments and second to accept sweet tastes and reject sour and bitter tastes. Then, as individuals, we each evolve in our own unique universe of tastes (to each his tastes!). This is our only hereditary baggage, which is by no means negligible, but which, in any case, will be profoundly modified, modulated, and broadened by social and cultural learning experiences.

3

The Taste
Preferences of
Children

After that long but necessary foray into the physiology
of tastes and flavors, let us return to the essential thing,
that is, taste-pleasure and food preferences. This chapter
will attempt to describe what children—the youngest as well as the
oldest, girls as well as boys, from everywhere in the world—like
or do not like, consume or do not consume. We will also try to
answer this question: can these tastes be explained as a function of
food criteria or different classes of food?

Children and Their Food Choices

Do children exhibit shared preferences and aversions? Or, on the
contrary, does each display specific tastes according to individual
sensory sensitivity?

Contrary to all expectations, very few studies attempt to describe children's tastes. Moreover, those that do focus primarily on adolescent populations. Thus, we can speak only of broad tendencies in children's taste, keeping in mind that the data, even when concordant, is not sufficient for drawing definitive conclusions.

Two kinds of studies exist. First, there are ones that survey attitudes. Subjects are presented with a list of foods, which may be short or long. As in a poll, they are then asked to give their opinion of each, that is, a hedonic assessment expressed, for example, as "I like very much," "I am indifferent," "I do not like," or even "I'm not familiar." The evaluation criteria vary according to the studies. The second kind of study observes the subjects' behavior, not their statements. They are presented actual foods and the quantity of the product they consume is measured.

In the first case (the opinion poll), there are four studies that allow us to broaden our discussion. In the second (observed consumption), only one study is available, though it is very interesting because it focuses on a large number of day-care children's meals. Let us try to compare the data resulting from these different studies. Let us try first to distinguish favorite foods, those that produced the greatest consensus with regard to acceptance, and then "outsider" foods, those rejected by the largest numbers.

Favorite Foods

The first survey, done by French researchers Matty Chiva and Claude Fischler in 1986, polled 321 French children, distributed over eight areas according to socioprofessional categories and divided into three age groups: four to seven years, eleven to twelve years, and seventeen to eighteen years. The children assessed a list of ninety-six foods on a hedonic scale with four levels: I like very much, I like, I do not like, and I do not like at all.

Most significantly, the study showed that the twenty foods on the list were appreciated by a very great number of children: from 85 to 66 percent of them claimed to "like very much" these foods. Moreover, the idea that preferences are the subject of strong consensus is confirmed again in a study conducted by Chiva and Baudier in 1990. The researchers asked a group of 882 adolescents, ages twelve to eighteen, coming from eleven French counties, to indicate their preferences on a list of 226 foods, assessed on a scale with three levels: I like, I am indifferent, and I do not like. The twenty most appreciated foods were chosen by 94 to 83 percent of the adolescents. The percentages are higher than in the Chiva and Fischler study because the subjects were asked not "Do you like this very much?" but simply "Do you like this?" Inevitably, the latter will produce a higher positive response. Another indication of consensus is that 67 percent of the foods were appreciated by more than half of the group, thirty-five foods by more than 80 percent of the group, and four foods by more than 90 percent.

These strong percentages, repeated in both the studies, corroborate the idea of the existence of consensus in children's preferences, shared by the great majority. Now, of course, comes the question: what are those favorite foods?

The favorite foods appearing in both studies are red fruits (strawberries, cherries, and raspberries among them), french fries, chocolate or chocolate bars, ice cream, chicken, yogurt, red meat, apricots, and oranges. We must also add fruit juices, crêpes, pasta, an array of fruits (peaches, melons, clementines, grapes, pears, bananas, and apples), quiche, cakes, pastries, white bread, fruit compote, crackers, butter, rice, mashed potatoes, and petit-suisse, a kind of sweet dessert cream cheese.

Moreover, all these results confirm those of a study recently conducted in France by the Kellogg Company that involved 997 children, nine to eleven years old. Of the forty-eight foods offered, only five were preferred by a sufficient percentage of the children to put them on equal footing with the foods on the top-twenty list: pizza, Nutella (a chocolate-hazelnut spread), candy, sandwiches, and Coca-Cola.

Finally, taking into account the disparity in the methods of these three studies, and the decade that passed between the first one and the last, the fact that quite similar results were obtained is an indication of their accuracy and consistency. We can extract from this table a kind of common denominator in matters of children's and adolescents' food tastes. At the top of the list are sweet foods, such as fruit, pastry, ice cream, and candy, and certain simple salty foods, for instance, starches like french fries, pasta, rice, bread, and pizza, and finally certain meats, especially steak and chicken. Notice that these foods in general are satisfying because of their high fat or carbohydrate content and offer little in the way of strong flavors.

Outsider Foods

The percentages for the twenty foods most often rejected are lower than those reflecting preferences. Thus, a greater consensus exists on favorite foods (up to 90 percent) than on least favorite foods (up to only 51 percent in the study by Fischler and Chiva, for example). Nevertheless, these numbers allow us to trace the parameters of a relative consensus in the expression of children's distastes for variety meats (liver, brains, tripe, kidneys, and beef tongue), most vegetables (cooked endive, cooked tomatoes, celery, cabbage, cauliflower, green pepper, spinach, turnips, and zucchini), and finally certain products that have very strong flavors or actively stimulate the trigeminal nerve (olives, strong cheeses, onions, and black pepper).

We must pay special attention to the problem of vegetables, as it greatly concerns parents. Often rightly but sometimes wrongly, they generally hold that children must eat vegetables—all vegetables. Yet there are other studies that confirm this very marked aversion to vegetables among children, especially the very young. A study conducted by Liliane Hanse in 1994 showed that the foods most often cited by mothers describing the food aversions of their children between the ages of two and ten were spinach, cauliflower, green beans, green salad, endive, mushrooms, and peas (and fish and liver must be added to that list). A study done by Vincent Boggio in 1992 involving the observation of choices made by children in day-care centers, in a self-serve situation, indicates that no vegetable dish made the list of products most often chosen.

But this unfavorable image of vegetables must be qualified. First of all, the distaste for them diminishes with age. Thus, more than 50 percent of adolescents come to appreciate green salad, cooked tomatoes, corn, radishes, raw carrots, green beans, peas, mushrooms, cucumbers, avocados, vegetable soup, artichokes, and asparagus.

Moreover, vegetables are certainly less appreciated than most other foods, but they are not necessarily the subject of a consensus of rejection. A significant variability among individuals appeared here that was not evident for fruits, for example. Thus, for cherries, 94 percent of children liked them, versus only 1 percent who did not like them. Whereas when we look at beets, 49 percent of day-care children chose them, as opposed to 15 percent who rejected them.

TWENTY FAVORITE FOODS IN TWO STUDIES

Study	Fischler and Chiva (1986)		Chiva and Baudier (1990)	
Number of Subjects	321 children and adolescents (4–18 years)		882 adolescents (12–18 years)	
Number of Foods	96		226	
Scale Used	5 points (++/+/−/−−/?)		4 points (+/0/−/?)	
Rank	% of "I love" responses		% of "I like" responses	
1	cherries	85*	fruit juice	94*
2	strawberries	85*	red fruits	93*
3	chocolate	85*	crêpes	93
4	french fries	84*	french fries	90*
5	raspberries	82*	peach, nectarine	90
6	ice cream	81*	quiche	89
7	chicken	78*	melon	89
8	yogurt	77*	clementines	89
9	pasta	77	cake	89
10	grapes	74	ice cream	89*
11	crackers	71	croissant, danish	88
12	butter	71	white bread	88
13	rice	70	chicken	87*
14	red meat	69*	orange	86*
15	mashed potatoes	68	yogurt with fruit	86*
16	apricot	68*	apricot	85*
17	petit-suisse	68	fruit compote	85
18	banana	68	chocolate bar	85*
19	apple	67	pear	85
20	orange	66*	hamburger	83*

*items included in both studies

We must thus stress the fact of strong differences among subjects with regard to their dislikes for this or that vegetable. To qualify still further, we must repeat that certain culinary preparations noticeably alter the assessment of products. In the study done by Boggio on the choices of day-care children, the number of times a dish was chosen by the children varied as much as one to four times according to the way it was prepared. For cauliflower, for example, 51 percent of children chose it among dishes when it was presented au gratin, as opposed to 36 percent if it was steamed and 15 percent if it was prepared in a salad.

To summarize, we can agree that taste preferences specific to children exist, as Fischler and Chiva thus define them: "the acceptance of a realm of foods known and appreciated by the majority of children and adolescents, beyond distinctions of sex, social or geographical origin, to the detriment of other rejected foods." In general, children appreciate products of simple composition that have a sweet taste and a fatty texture, are mildly flavored, and are satisfying to the appetite.

These parameters of children's and adolescents' tastes could explain in part why children tend to reject vegetables—which especially fail to satisfy the appetite. But other explanations have been proposed, which we will explore presently.

Different Kinds of Distaste

What motivates individuals to accept or reject this or that category of products? To answer this question, Paul Rozin, one of the prominent American psychologists studying taste, proposed a classification system based on numerous interviews with American adults that was then validated with children. In terms of rejection or acceptance, the author was able to establish three broad categories of motivations. Reexamined with regard to rejections, this classification results in the definition of sensory distastes, cognitive distastes, and associative distastes—or "distaste," "disgust," and "danger."

Sensory Distastes

The first category is the one that permits us to distinguish between foods that taste "good" and those that taste "bad." Here, the "taste of" (flavor) is at the origin of the "taste for" (taste-pleasure or displeasure). Thus, anyone might say, "I accept this food because I find it good on the sensory level" or "I reject it because it produces disagreeable sensations" (visual, olfactory, or in the mouth). Sensory rejection can, at this point, be strong enough to transmute into true "distaste."

In a general sense, we find sweet products on the side of acceptance, since people are programmed to accept them, and bitter or spicy products on the side of rejection. This is especially true for children. But learning allows these reactions inscribed in the organism to be overcome. That is why, in adulthood, true lovers of coffee, beer, and spicy dishes develop.

But there also exist products known as segmentors. That is, they do not produce consensus; certain people accept them and others reject them, even at the youngest ages. Let us look at some typical examples on the side of distaste. We have already discussed the strong rejection of cauliflower by people who are tasters of PTC, and its possible acceptance among nontasters. Similarly,

TWENTY OUTSIDER FOODS IN TWO STUDIES

Study	Fischler and Chiva (1986)		Chiva and Baudier (1990)	
Number of Subjects	321 children and adolescents (4–18 years)		882 adolescents (12–18 years)	
Number of Foods	96		226	
Scale Used	5 points (++/+/-/--/?)		4 points (+/0/-/?)	
Rank	% of "I do not like" responses		% of "that disgusts me" responses	
1	milk skin	51	brains	57*
2	brains	45*	tripe	53
3	black olives	41*	liver	43*
4	pepper	36	oysters	42
5	garlic	36	blood sausage	40
6	onion	35	wine	39
7	strong cheese	31*	kidneys	35
8	green olives	30	white sausage	35
9	sparkling water	29	beer	34
10	celery	28*	chestnut cream	34
11	cooked tomato	26	beef tongue	33
12	green pepper	25*	Roquefort cheese	32*
13	spinach	25*	cooked endive	31
14	liver	24*	cabbage	28*
15	warm milk	24	strong spices	27
16	cold milk	21	turnips	26
17	mustard	21	green pepper	26*
18	zucchini	19	creamed celery	26*
19	cauliflower	17*	spinach	25*
20	corn	17	black olives	25*

*items included in both studies

cheese is appreciated by some but provokes rejection among others, even if its presence is imperceptible, as when it is hidden in a prepared sauce. Well before others, the rejecters of cheese perceive its odor, no matter what the quantity, and it is the odor that produces their sensory distaste. Among children, fish, green olives, and carbonated drinks also divide the population into lovers and nonlovers.

Thus we see that the distribution of foods according to this first criterion, of good or bad flavor, is more or less general to the population. Nevertheless, it remains the essential factor in preferences and aversions among children. In other words, if young children are asked to indicate dishes that they appreciate and those they find displeasing, a good estimation of 80 percent of their actual food consumption can be inferred. But the strongest correlation remains between what is rejected and what is not consumed.

This correlation between preference and consumption is not nearly as evident among adults, who let other considerations enter into their choices beside purely sensory ones. Adults can appreciate chocolate enormously but consume it in very small quantities. Children, on the other hand, when given the choice, will limitlessly consume those products they find extremely pleasant in the mouth. The difference comes from the fact that adults refer not solely to sensory pleasure but also to many other factors relating to the representation of foods. For example, is this dish expensive or inexpensive? Will it make me fat? Is it consumed in summer or winter? Morning or evening? These are some of the many cognitive or situational factors that we will discuss next.

Cognitive Distastes

The second broad category of motivations concerns intellectual or cultural representations of foods, which render them more or less acceptable. Within this vast group, Paul Rozin identified a particularly interesting subcategory that he called cognitive distastes, or "disgusts," which are differentiated from sensory distastes. Rejection based on cognitive distaste takes place not as a function of the taste of the food but as a function of its nature, its origin, or the associations it brings up.

Animal products are often good examples of cognitive distastes. If variety meats tend to be rejected, it is mainly because of their origin and their function. If the idea of consuming a cockroach provokes strong disgust in us, it is because this animal is associated with filth and unhealthy places.

This last example is governed by a purely cultural representation. In other countries, especially in Latin America, the cockroach evokes entirely different images. It is a food greatly appreciated for its crunchiness and its high nutritional value. In the same way, the rejection Anglo-Saxons demonstrate toward snails, frogs, and horse meat derives from cultural images. From early childhood, such foods of animal origin are described to them as inedible.

Within a single culture, other types of representation, more insidious but just as powerful in shaping our food tastes, hold sway. Let us consider the example of garlic. Parents are informed by the media that lactating women must not ingest dishes with garlic or their newborns will refuse to drink their breast milk. Later on, these same parents who make pureed vegetables for their babies do not dare enliven the dish with a clove of garlic. Questioned about their behavior, they declare this plant unsuitable for children, reserved for use in cooking for adults. Nevertheless, most young children easily accept the flavor of garlic. It is only later that they may manifest some opposition.

Is this later rejection the cause or the effect of the image of garlic as an "adult product"? If it were the cause, children beyond a certain age would no longer be able to accept the strong flavor of garlic. Thus, parents would have an accurate image of this condiment, although they would be overgeneralizing it to include very young children. If it were the effect, those same children would not be able to appreciate garlic because their parents never offered it to them. In this way, a kind of vicious circle is created: the less a food is offered, the less willing children are to accept it, since the product remains unfamiliar and thus unacceptable.

This category of rejections, dependent on a whole complex of images, is the one that least concerns young children. As we will see, cognitive distastes rarely appear before the age of three. Associative distastes, on the other hand, can be the subject of very early learning experiences.

Associative Distastes

In addition to sensory distastes and cognitive distastes, there is a final category that I will call associative or conditioned distastes. This is a matter of rejections associated with the consequences of ingesting a certain food, a mechanism that alerts us to "danger."

The example of aversions best represents distastes associated with postingestion effects. This involves rejection resulting from a unique experience with a certain food. Here is a scenario that perfectly illustrates the phenomenon: eat a new food and contract intestinal flu a few hours later; you will no doubt experience a lasting distaste for that food. The food is mistakenly associated with the gastric displeasure, and from this association results a very powerful aversion that is difficult to overcome.

This phenomenon is well known in cancer treatment services. In effect, patients undergoing chemotherapy come to develop numerous aversions resulting from associations between dishes they eat and the intestinal upset they suffer following medical treatments. To overcome this added discomfort, certain facilities introduce new foods into their menus. The aversions then become centered on these new foods, and the usual repertoire of consumption remains unaffected, so that the patient can eat normally upon returning home.

Finally, let us note that the association between food and gastric troubles is sometimes justified. Such is the case if the food has gone bad or if it presents a certain degree of toxicity. Thus, eating bad squid just once can be enough to produce a long-lasting aversion to seafood.

In contrast to what happens in the case of aversions, the effects of ingestion can prove to be positive. The phenomenon of preferences acquired through the process of satisfying one's appetite is a perfect illustration of this. We have seen that satiating products, which quickly appease the sensations of hunger by filling the stomach, are particular favorites of children. This observation prompts the following questions: Are these foods preferred because of their power to appease hunger? And if so, does that mean that children know how to recognize the satiating effects of foods?

Studies have effectively shown that infants know how to adapt the quantity of fluid they ingest according to its caloric concentration. The more diluted the milk, the greater the quantity they will drink; the more concentrated it is, the richer, and the higher its caloric content, the less of it they will consume. This proves that newborns know how to recognize their sensations of satiation. When they are hungry, they learn to associate what they drink with the capacity of that liquid to satisfy them. But this type of learning does not happen with a single try; many repetitions are necessary.

Leann Birch, a prominent American taste psychologist, conducted experiments on older children, ages three to five. She formed three groups and familiarized them with one type of cracker. The first group had available to them a cracker with a low caloric content; the second group had the same cracker, with the same flavor, but with a higher caloric content; the third had a cracker with a very high caloric content. She had the children eat these crackers a certain number of times, always giving the same type to each group. At the end of the experiment, she offered them all the same cracker with a medium caloric level.

Birch observed that the children familiar with a lower caloric intensity consumed a greater quantity of the medium crackers than those familiar with a high caloric intensity. Thus, the children had learned to associate the taste, or the flavor of the food, with a certain satiating effect. Those who had had the hypocaloric cracker knew that it was necessary to eat many of them to feel satisfied. Even when offered a cracker with a medium and, for them, higher caloric level, they continued to eat more. Those who had had the hypercaloric cracker had learned to eat a little to be satisfied. But if the children continued to be given crackers with the medium caloric content, they adapted all over again.

Birch conducted a second experiment on this topic, mixing children and adults. She offered them as appetizers, ad libitum, a whole array of products usually consumed before going to the table. She then observed their behavior during the meal. She noted that the children, much more so than the adults, modified the quantity of food they ingested at the table in relation to what they had eaten beforehand. This seems to indicate that children, in the end, regulate their appetites better than adults.

These different studies show that children are particularly sensitive to the more or less satiating quality of foods. Their repeated experiences with a food allow them to establish a link between its flavor and its ingestive effects. That could explain children's preference for products that quickly appease sensations of hunger (starchy foods especially) and, conversely, their tendency to reject vegetables.

Let us recall that sensory or cognitive motivations can be the grounds for rejecting vegetables as well. In the first case, it is their bad taste; the disagreeable flavor of a vegetable can justify its rejection. In the second case, it is a negative image, as with a dreary product linked to coercion, that sets off the reaction.

Nevertheless, let us take advantage of the example of vegetables to repeat that the sensory, cognitive, or associative nature of our distastes can make its presence felt on the side of preferences. From this perspective, vegetables might be perceived as products that taste good, are good to think about, and are good for our health. We will see that the relatively positive or negative image of vegetables is not the same for everyone. Most notably, it differentiates the youngest subjects from the oldest, as well as the girls from the boys.

Do Girls and Boys, Big and Little, Have Similar Taste Preferences?

Earlier, we described the taste preferences of children in general. Now, we will consider whether these tastes evolve with age or according to gender, as a function of the nature of tastes and distastes.

The Effect of Age on Food Preferences

The question of the evolution of children's tastes with age can be examined especially through the study by Fischler and Chiva, who distinguished three age groups. The researchers noted that certain foods were particularly rejected by the youngest children, those between the ages of four and seven years. It was primarily a matter of foods with strong flavors—vinaigrette dressing, cornichon pickles, black pepper, garlic, black olives, onion, mustard, and grapefruit. By way of example, garlic and onion enjoyed approximately the same evolution: less than 20 percent of four- to seven-year-olds appreciated them, as opposed to 60 percent of seventeen- and eighteen-year-olds.

The study by Fischler and Chiva also supports the idea that vegetables become less and less objectionable as children grow older. Ton Nu, who did a survey among adolescents ten to twenty years old, confirms this observation. Endive, spinach, and cabbage, which are hardly favorites in this period of life, are nevertheless the subject of greater acceptance beginning at the age of twelve years.

With regard to populations of young children, Boggio notes that beginning at two years of age children less and less often choose dishes made from cucumber, tomato, zucchini, leek, and salsify. In the study by Liliane Hanse that involved children between the ages of two and ten, the category of vegetables declines in preference rankings until the age of seven, at which point it begins to rise and appears to stabilize around the twentieth position; it is least appreciated between the ages of five and a half and seven. Similarly, soup occupies the thirteenth position in the preference rankings of children younger than two and a half; beginning at four years, it is no longer among the favorite foods.

PREFERENCE RANKINGS FOR THE CATEGORY OF VEGETABLES IN THE STUDY BY HANSE (1994)

Age Group	Rank
less than 2.5 years	31
2.5 years to 3 years, 11 months	17
4 years to 5 years, 5 months	24
5.5 years to 6 years, 11 months	45
7 years to 8 years, 5 months	16
8.5 years to 10 years	18

From observations like these involving the rejection of vegetables and foods with pronounced flavors, it is tempting to conclude that sensory distastes diminish with age. On the other hand, we can note an inverse tendency for cognitive distastes.

On this subject, let us cite a series of novel experiments conducted by Paul Rozin. For example, working with a population of American children and adults, this researcher proposed stirring a drink of hot chocolate with a plastic comb that the subjects were assured had never been used. While the children generally agreed to consume the drink stirred in this way, the idea of contact produced a strong cognitive distaste among the adults; most of them refused to sample it. In the same way, presented with a meal in a dog bowl, also verified to be clean and never-before used, subjects were observed to quite categorically refuse to consume the food, and in ever greater numbers according to their ages.

This is explained by the fact that the cognitive system for processing information becomes more complex with age. Whereas the youngest children never imagine that the object of disgust could contaminate the product to be consumed, for adults contamination is much more significant, threatening, and an impediment to their behavior. Thus it appears that, contrary to what we might believe, magical thinking increases in certain areas as humans age.

These examples are caricatures of how cognitive distastes intensify with age. They bring us back, however, to the more common rejection of variety meats. Indeed, the study by Fischler and Chiva, for example, does find animal by-products to be rejected more often by adolescents than by young children.

In conclusion, let us reiterate that there is an inverse evolution of cognitive distastes and sensory distastes as a function of age. As they get older, children demonstrate increasing rejection of certain foods with negative images (variety meats) and increasing acceptance of other foods with stronger flavors (certain vegetables and seasoning products). The rejection of vegetables in particular begins at about two years, reaches its height between five and seven years, and noticeably diminishes beginning at twelve years. But also beginning at that age, a difference between girls' and boys' preferences becomes apparent.

The Effect of Gender on Food Preferences

Beginning with puberty, which corresponds to specific ages for girls and for boys, differences in tastes according to gender appear, differences practically nonexistent before that time. We observe that girls demonstrate a much more pronounced taste for raw and cooked vegetables, while boys are more attracted to animal products, especially meat, butter, and sometimes milk; both like sweetened drinks.

These changes can be explained on two levels. First of all—and this may be the most plausible explanation—these modifications in behavior are really responses to aesthetic concerns, which are very clearly different for girls and for boys. Young women pay much greater attention to the problem of gaining weight. But another fact, less well known, can also explain certain gender differentiations in taste. Beginning with menstruation, girls experience a hormonal change that makes them much more sensitive to the sweet taste. Thus, for example, the fact that adolescent girls put much less sugar in their cereal than boys do may indeed be explained by girls' greater attention to their figures, but it may also be because the sweet taste is suddenly much stronger in their mouths.

Another gender difference beginning at puberty concerns the degree of food selectivity. Girls prove more picky and reject a greater number of foods than boys do. Here we can invoke a supposedly female trait: women may be "more picky." But we can also look for explanation in the fact that in general girls know how to express their choices and their aversions much more clearly than boys. From this perspective, they are being not more picky but more definitive in their choices, more self-assured, and less fickle.

Whatever the case, these differences in taste preferences between girls and boys remain minor in relationship to the impressive consensus that emerges from a single and unique culture.

Is Taste Here the Same As Elsewhere?

As we have seen in the studies by Fischler and Chiva (1986) and Chiva and Baudier (1990), discussed earlier in this chapter, French children appear to agree in their appreciation of a certain number of foods and their rejection of others. Are their choices similar to those of children from other cultures, forming one large community of shared preferences and rejections that mark the parameters of the universal taste preferences of children? Or, on the contrary, does each culture possess its own food repertoire, and beyond that, its own cuisine, composed of specific rules and images?

The Tastes of France and North America

The many limitations of scientific methodology do not allow for a relevant comparison between the taste preferences of subjects belonging to different cultures. The ideal would be to conduct a study in which subjects from different cultures were asked to sample identical tastes; their reactions would then be observed. In that way, differences in the hedonic assessment of products could be observed, as well as differences in the perception of intensity and quality.

But alas, such studies are not available. We must thus settle for comparing surveys conducted in one country with those conducted in another. But an additional problem then arises because certain foods appreciated in one country may not exist in other countries. So it remains very risky to compare, for example, Westerners with Africans or Indians, as their food repertoires are so very far removed from one another's.

We could compare the food choices of French and American populations, because foods common to both civilizations do exist. Nevertheless, many differences remain. For example, if we compare the studies conducted in France to American studies, what can we say about how culture affects French appreciation for dinner rolls and strawberry shortcake? Conversely, what can we say about American appreciation for crêpes, croissants, and petit-suisse?

It follows then that only the foods common to both cultures

can be the subject of comparison. And this statement must be further qualified. If we want to compare the ranking of preference for ice cream in France and the United States, are we taking into consideration the creamy, very sweet ice creams that exist in the United States, or the less creamy, more sharply flavored sorbet-type ice creams that are very much the reference for French subjects? There again, it is not a strict comparison because the products offer obvious sensory differences.

For the United States, the two most important surveys are somewhat dated, since they were done in the 1970s and '80s, polling soldiers and American students. The foods most appreciated by students and the American military were as follows: ice cream, roast turkey, dinner rolls, roast chicken, steak, a whole series of desserts, french fries, and milk. We may note that, despite a certain regional variability, American preferences are largely defined by the sweet taste and proteins of animal origin. Thirty percent of the favorite foods were desserts; another 30 percent were meats. These surveys also point to the existence of shared tastes in the food preferences of American adolescents and young adults.

Beginning with this data, we may ask whether American preferences are comparable to those noted in French studies. Identical tendencies appear in the studies done on both sides of the Atlantic. The two youth populations have clear preferences for certain foods like french fries, pasta, chicken, red meat, and some fruit products. On the side of rejection, we can note that the class of vegetables is rejected both in France and in the United States, especially in terms of cauliflower, spinach, and cooked tomatoes, as is the class of variety meats.

But other products give the impression of an intercultural

differentiation. Milk, for example, which does not make the list of favorite foods in France (garnering between 50 and 60 percent positive responses, according to the studies, as opposed to 31 percent negative), was appreciated by 92 percent of the subjects in one American study.

As for hamburgers, 88 percent of Americans appreciate them, as opposed to about 70 percent of the French population. However, if we focus on the ranking of preferences, the cultural difference appears more clearly: hamburgers, which occupy the 15th ranking for 207 food preferences in an American study, occupy only the 175th ranking for 226 food preferences in the French study by Chiva and Baudier from 1990.

Despite the similarity in French and American food repertoires, the cultural environment shapes the food preferences and rejections specific to each culture. Shared tendencies between the two Western cultures do appear, however. French and American children both seem to appreciate filling products and to reject vegetables. It is true that food fulfills a vital and universal function: it provides nourishment. Nevertheless, culture shapes the pleasure we take in eating. And beyond tastes, the cuisine unique to each culture is rooted in the culture itself.

The Concept of Cuisine

Cultural learning has especially interested sociologists, such as Claude Fischler in France. In his work *L'homnivore,* he gives the following definition of cuisine: "an ensemble of ingredients and foodstuffs used in the preparation of food, or, in a broader sense, rules and representations associated with them that are shared by the members of a single culture or a group within that culture." Thus, the term "cuisine" designates, first, an array of foods and, second, not a series of recipes but an array of habits governed by rules and images specific to a cultural group.

The cultural system for foods operates in concentric circles. The widest circle is universal. It represents the whole of potentially edible foods, that is, all the foods consumed on the face of the planet. The second is the whole of comestible foods in a given culture, the ensemble that encompasses horse meat and snails in France and the cockroach in South American countries. Those products are appreciated in one place but are the subject of strong cognitive distaste elsewhere. That is the difference between "edible" and "comestible."

Within the category of comestible, there is a subgroup made up of a culture's repertoire of customary, familiar foods. This includes foods eaten quite commonly within a specific culture, having sensory images known to all its members. The habitual repertoire is particularly appreciated by children, who find stable references there.

Within this repertoire of familiar foods exists a very specialized group consisting of two subgroups. First, the basic foods, consumed at nearly every meal; bread in France and rice in Asian countries are good examples of this. Second, the elements of flavor, that is, sapid combinations very commonly used as seasonings within a single culture. Examples are the combination of olive oil, garlic, and tomato in Mediterranean countries; the combination of lemon juice, peppers, and grated carrots in southeast Asia; and the tomato–hot-pepper combination in Mexican cuisine.

Culinary representations and rules, not just foods, define the cuisine specific to each culture. We understand representations to mean more or less arbitrary but fixed cultural images for products.

We have already mentioned the primary rule, the rule of comestibility, which defines the horse as a food in France but as noncomestible elsewhere. We have also discussed products that convey an image of being meant or not meant for children. The decision is of a cultural order: in the United States, hot peppers would never be offered to children, whereas young Mexicans, provided repeated (and progressively hotter!) experiences with peppers, would not know what to do without them.

Fischler particularly emphasizes the fact that a certain number of very complex rules govern our way of feeding ourselves. He classifies these rules into two subsystems. First, the rules termed "intrinsic," which, within a single meal, determine the organization of the various foods and their associations. For example, Mexican cuisine employs avocado extensively in main courses, whereas in other countries it would be considered a fruit and consumed for dessert. Likewise, the rule of having sweet-salty combinations is part of cultural custom in Scandinavian countries, but it is rarely accepted in France, where only a special occasion, such as a holiday meal, would give license to that combination, used, for example, in duck with orange sauce.

The rules termed "extrinsic" involve the way meals fit into the context of the day. These are more temporal rules, like the timetable for eating. In the United States one generally dines at about six o'clock, in France at about eight o'clock, and in Spain at about ten o'clock.

Experiments have demonstrated that these cultural rules are linked to our preferences and rejections; in fact, they tend to dictate them. Birch conducted an experiment among children, ages three to five, and adults. She asked them to specify their preferences for a series of foods that, according to the rules, are considered breakfast foods or dinner foods. For example, hot chocolate and pizza were on the list. The novelty in her approach was that she measured preferences for the morning and for the evening. She noted that beginning at age four children will say they prefer to consume hot chocolate in the morning rather than in the evening, and pizza in the evening rather than in the morning. This clearly shows the impact of cultural internalization on food preferences and rejections.

Even though they are arbitrary, these rules and images have a great influence on our food behavior. Moreover, simply breaking with these cultural habits can prompt reactions of distrust and rejection, especially with regard to unfamiliar products. However, the modern food industry is gradually equalizing cultural differences by offering the same products everywhere. Just five years ago, for example, couscous could not have been considered part of our familiar repertoire. Today, it is recognized by a great number of people around the world and is sold in almost every U.S. supermarket.

Thus we are at this moment witnessing a phenomenon of globalization. Cultural customs, rules, and representations are becoming less and less powerful. The consequences are twofold: positive for the opening of the world that globalization represents, and negative for what constitutes an undeniable loss of cultural identity.

In effect, cuisines serve a dual function. The first is to shape our cultural identity. For Rozin, the best way to predict the cultural identity of an individual is to ask what he eats. The second function of these cultural habits is to dictate to us what we ought to consume and in what context, thus helping us avoid ever having to make difficult choices. In a certain way, they mitigate the anxiety of incorporation, experienced by omnivores and especially by children, which we will discuss in relationship to food neophobia.

4
The Phenomenon of Food Neophobia

What do we mean by food neophobia? Literally, it signifies a fear of novelty in the area of food. Subjects feel fear at tasting any new and therefore unknown food. This fear is common. We have all shown reluctance at one time or another to put into our mouths a food we have never tasted.

Scientific literature began to take an interest in this issue in the 1970s, first in the observation of rats. Conducted in the United States, these experiments showed that when presented with new foods, rats exhibit distrustful behavior that takes on different forms according to age: An adult would confidently taste the product, but in a very small quantity, and it would taste it again only after a long waiting period and on the condition that no problems arose following its ingestion. On the other hand, young rats, even if they were famished, would wait for the adults to taste the food before helping themselves.

Following these studies on rats, three branches of the human sciences further examined the question of food neophobia: sociology, child psychology, and comparative psychology, which involves the differences between individuals.

The Sociological Approach

It was Paul Rozin himself, the American psychologist, who launched these experiments on rats. Subsequently, he attempted to transpose this concept to sociology. In France the sociologist Claude Fischler followed up on Rozin's work and notably enlarged upon it. Even though the two researchers have developed the concept of neophobia in two different ways, their thinking on it finally remains quite similar.

The Anxiety of Incorporation

For Paul Rozin, food neophobia among humans is due essentially to our condition as omnivores. Human beings must consume a wide repertoire of foods—and introduce much variety into that repertoire—in order to meet purely physiological needs. Thus, there is a universal genetic inscription that urges humans to seek out new products. This pursuit of novelty, necessary to survival, is called neophilia.

Paradoxically, it is accompanied by neophobia, reinforced by an anxiety of incorporation, that is, a fear of introducing into oneself unknown products. On this level, the mouth truly represents a kind of border checkpoint between the outside and inside worlds, through which it is difficult for products with potentially harmful effects to enter.

These harmful effects are located on two planes. First, we wit-

ness a fear of poisoning, of dying from ingesting products dangerous to human health. And even though, at the start of the third
millennium, our industrialized societies generally offer us products that are subject to quite strict safety standards, all the excite-
ment surrounding the "mad cow" outbreaks, to consider only one
example, reminds us that neither man nor beast is ever safe from
poisoned food. Thus this phobia features a certain rationality.

But there is also a much more symbolic anxiety, more closely
related to the magical thinking that coexists side by side with rational thinking, even among scientific researchers of great renown.
An experiment conducted by Rozin illustrates this magical anxiety
of incorporation with regard to food.

He told his second-year psychology students that he was
conducting a study on racial prejudices and distributed to them
a handout describing all the common practices of an imaginary
ethnic group: holiday customs, traditional dress, and, of course, a
few items on their eating habits. But, unbeknownst to the students,
the text was presented in two versions. Only one sentence varied.
In the first version, the ethnic group was described as consuming
sea turtles and hunting wild boar for their tusks. In the second, the
ethnic group was described as eating wild boar and hunting sea
turtles for their shells.

The students were asked to read this text and then respond to
a questionnaire on the characteristics of individuals belonging to
this ethnic group. Different personality traits were thus measured.
Rozin analyzed the questionnaires and compared the responses of
the "turtle" and "wild boar" groups. The results indicated very
little significant difference between the two groups, except that the
first group described the individuals of this ethnicity as peaceful
and good swimmers, while the second group described them as

warlike and fast runners. The psychologist thus observed an irrational belief according to which the symbolic properties of foods transform us, indicative of magical thinking in the area of food.

A great number of food advertisements operate according to this principle of magical thinking: "Drink water X and you will experience psychic harmony," "Eat yogurt Y and you will become pure," or even "Munch on a lion and you will develop superhuman strength." This belief also appears in some of our maxims, according to which meat lovers are aggressive, whereas consumers of certain vegetables, turnips for example, prove to be passive and cowardly. It may explain why some adults do not offer foods with strong flavors to children. If children are considered to embody sweetness and gentleness, giving them too-strong tastes could contribute to their too-rapid development. Let us remember that primitive societies do not hold exclusive rights to magical thinking, which in some ways is opposed to rational thinking. It is alive and well in all societies, even the most industrialized ones in our modern Western world.

According to Rozin, the anxiety of incorporation (rational or magical) is present in all species that must make choices in the area of food. Neophobia is the counterpart of neophilia, the need to seek out novelty that characterizes omnivorous species. This fundamental contradiction is designated as the "omnivore's paradox." All human beings must learn to reconcile their need for novelty, a physiological necessity, and their fear of the unknown, whether rationally or irrationally founded.

UCOs: Unidentified Comestible Objects

For his part, Claude Fischler considers neophobia to revolve around what he, in his colorful fashion, calls "OCNIs" or, in English,

"UCOs": unidentified comestible objects. This would be a matter of unfamiliar foods, whether they are part of a foreign cuisine or an outcome of innovation. For Fischler, UCOs are essentially the result of modern food production. He developed the idea that current food production and distribution systems tend to reinforce the unidentifiable nature of most of our foods.

Over the past several decades (about fifty years), a certain number of sociological changes have resulted in the fact that food preparation is gradually being replaced by "factory cuisine." Among these changes, we can cite the establishment of wide distribution networks, the development of urban life, and the desire to limit the time devoted to household activities, especially the preparation of meals. Thus "in-house" production has become the exception and the distance separating the production site and our plates has steadily grown, so much so that modern eaters consume principally quasi-manufactured, "denaturalized" foodstuffs, of which they know neither the history nor the origin.

The convenience of industrial products is undeniable. Nevertheless, the omnivore faces many questions with regard to this "ready-to-eat" food. What does our food contain? Where did it come from? How has it been processed? Who has touched it? And so on. The interest directed at the brand, the label, the place of origin, and the packaging may be an attempt to reidentify the product.

Modern eaters find themselves torn between two contradictory tendencies: the attraction to the convenience of factory-made foodstuffs and the doubts that they raise. This hesitancy is reinforced by the growing diversity of products available on the market. In becoming modern, the omnivore is led to make more and more choices. And these choices prove to be more and more individual because culture is losing its power to provide us with collective frameworks for consumption.

Neophobia, supported by the anxiety of incorporation, is well and truly universal. It affects Rozin's neophilic eater through the omnivore's paradox, and it affects Fischler's modern eater confronted with invading UCOs. In all times, humans reject the unknown because they need to know what they eat; they must be able to identify their foods. Thus young humans, in growing up, must be able to learn to recognize their foods.

The Developmental Approach

If it is not always easy to recognize the existence of a universal neophobia, all parents recognize the phenomenon of childhood neophobia. What child has not, in effect, shown disgust in the face of a new dish? How many children have not proven particularly selective in their food choices during some period in their lives?

If the phenomenon is so ubiquitous, let us consider it a necessary stage, normal in the development of the child. But this does not keep us from asking the real question: why do children prove to be particularly neophobic?

The Normal Stage of Food Selectivity

We know that familiarity is paramount in the food tastes of young children. In the late 1970s Leann Birch showed that two factors dominate in the preferences of children three to five years old: sweetness and the degree of familiarity. We have already seen that the preference for sweet among children is a very powerful innate factor. What matters is that familiarity plays as important a role in the acceptance of foods as sweet taste does. In general, observations show that the better known a food is, the more it is appreciated.

Following Birch, a few researchers have studied neophobia, which, according to them, corresponds to a "normal" stage in individual development in the statistical sense. In fact, neophobia affects the majority of children, who, at various times, reject new foods. We are still lacking statistical data on the subject because interest in it is only recent. The biggest study was done in France in 1994 by the psychologist Liliane Hanse. She surveyed nearly six hundred mothers with children between the ages of two and ten, using a questionnaire focusing on the changes in their children's eating behavior over the course of time.

The chief result of the study was to show that between two and ten years of age only 23 percent of children demonstrate no neophobic behavior. This means that only one child out of four will willingly taste a new food, without needing to be compelled in some way.

Childhood food neophobia can be witnessed through various behaviors such as those listed below. This list, proposed by Liliane Hanse, is organized according to frequency, from the behaviors most often observed to those most rarely observed.

A child older than two will sort out the various foods in a mixed dish. At any age, children will proceed to carefully examine the products. They will grimace, recalling the gusto-facial reflex produced by bitterness; they will turn the food over and over with their forks, sniff it, and then chew it for a long time, even if that prolongs the time they must keep it in their mouths before swallowing it.

Some children categorically refuse to taste a new food, often spitting it out if they do. Pushing away the plate or spoon, turning the head away, or even refusing to open the mouth are a number of ways small children (about two years old) manifest their neophobia.

The foods children refuse to taste—and fortunately they continue to accept others—are those with strong flavors and—surprise!—vegetables. When mothers were asked to list in descending order the foods they had the most trouble getting their children to accept, the list was as follows: spinach, cauliflower, vegetables in general, green beans, fish, green salad, meat, raw vegetables, endive, liver, mushrooms, and peas. This corroborates the existence of a children's taste preference that, in terms of rejections, centers especially on vegetables and strong-tasting products.

Beginning from these results, we can affirm that over the course of childhood, neophobia takes on a broader meaning. It is no longer just a matter of rejecting unknown foods but much more a matter of restricting the repertoire of consumption. Until they are two years old, the vast majority of children easily accept most foods. Beginning at two, vegetables, which were previously well accepted, are suddenly rejected. Thus, we must speak not of rejecting new foods—of neophobia—in the strict sense but of a decrease in the number of foods accepted.

However, it is between four and seven years that children prove to be the most neophobic. It is not that greater numbers of children this age manifest neophobia, but that this is the age when they demonstrate the greatest rigidity and categorically refuse to consume certain foods offered to them. After seven, and until about ten to eleven, we witness a lull in their neophobic behavior. They continue to be selective in their food choices, of course, but attempts to alter the context of consumption and various parental incentives can be successful, even with regard to vegetables.

These ages are the statistical average, and each child will find his or her own rhythm. Some will be more precocious; others will demonstrate almost no neophobia. To qualify this scenario once more, we must remember that the study involved indirect observation. Mothers were asked to remember the behavior of their children regarding food. It was not a matter of direct observation, whereby children would be confronted with new foods under the watchful eye of researchers who would witness and record in a precise, objective fashion their rejections.

While we wait for subsequent studies to confirm these results, we may well ask ourselves, as does every parent confronted with a child obstinately refusing some dish, why neophobia is particularly strong beginning at two to four years up until the age of seven.

How to Explain Neophobia in Children

Four major hypotheses have been proposed. The first, the one that parents, when asked, sometimes advance, is that neophobia may be nothing more or less than a demonstration of opposition to parents, which, moreover, can be observed in all areas. Thus, it may or may not correspond to a phase witnessed in practically all children. And it is true that without knowing it certain children confirm this hypothesis by eating much more willingly at school or with their playmates than when at home.

Seen from this perspective, neophobia could be a manifestation of the process of individuation that all children experience when they are about two to three years old, which consists of constructing for themselves an individual identity, distinct from that of their parents. For certain children, neophobia could also reflect a need to differentiate themselves from their siblings, as though

NEOPHOBIC BEHAVIORS AND APPEARANCE PERCENTAGES
AMONG CHILDREN TWO TO TEN

Behavior	Percentage of Children Who Exhibited Behavior
Sorting out mixed foods	56
Examining foods	45
Grimacing	31
Chewing for a long time	31
Turning food over and over with a fork	31
Refusing the food without tasting it	28
Spitting food out	25
Sniffing food	18
Other behaviors	18
Vomiting if forced to swallow food	12
Pushing away the plate or spoon	9
Turning the head away	8
Refusing to open the mouth	7

to say, "Of all my brothers and sisters, I am the most difficult when it comes to eating. Thus I am the center of attention during meals, while the others, being easier to feed, do not receive the same attention."

This hypothesis would explain why neophobia appears when it does, at about two to three years of age. However, it is not sufficient for explaining why opposition centers on unknown foods.

The second hypothesis, proposed by Chiva and Fischler, sees neophobia as a manifestation of the need for security at the age when children enter school. In fact, from ages two to three up until about age seven, we witness an intense learning period, sometimes experienced by children as unsettling. Thus, a child might seek a secure sector in the area of food. Also, children might reject certain foods they consider too adventurous and prove partial to stable, familiar references. This idea is corroborated by the fact that food, at all ages and in a universal fashion, is experienced as potentially dangerous.

The third hypothesis relates to the fact that children, beginning at about one and a half to two years, start to exhibit a certain autonomy, first in their behavior, since they are eating by themselves, and second in their food choices. They can more easily decide whether the product presented to them is known or unknown, and then perhaps refuse it. What matters is that at this age children are learning to make their first choices, to make decisions. Consequently, they find themselves confronting the anxiety of incorporation. It is up to them to decide whether they will incorporate a food, taking on the associated risks. Formerly their parents assumed this responsibility and thus spared them the torments of uncertainty. According to Patricia Pliner, young children's hesitations are reinforced by their lack of cultural reference points. Unlike adults, they are not conscious of the controls exerted by society to guarantee a certain level of safety in the area of food.

The last hypothesis, the one that I propose, involves the development of intellectual mechanisms in the child. In the area of cognition, Jean Piaget demonstrated that children exhibit great perceptive rigidity between the ages of two and seven (called the preoperations stage). If one part of an object changes, the object becomes totally new for them. They have difficulty integrating the different parts of an object into one thing. They will focus attention successively on its different dimensions—its size, color, and shape—without being able to conceive of them constituting a whole.

In the area of food, we can easily observe this by presenting a child with a familiar food, like the classic dish of mashed pota-toes. Just changing a single characteristic, for example, garnishing it with a bit of parsley and thus transforming the visual aspect, is enough to make the child see a new food, which then prompts neophobia and rejection.

In other words, this hypothesis holds that we witness a nor-mal stage of development of neophobia in children between two and seven years of age because the indications of novelty are more numerous at that age. For the child, changing a single quality in a familiar product is enough to transform it completely. In this stage of life, there exist as many new foods as there exist ways to present the same product.

As different as they appear, these four hypotheses—opposition to parents, a need for security, growing autonomy, and intellectual rigidity—are nevertheless not incompatible and can coexist on various levels in the explanation of neophobia. And if none of them has been verified by sufficiently numerous scientific stud-ies, there is nevertheless evidence that tends to corroborate the idea that children and adults have different definitions for what is new. In other words, children see novelty where it may not necessarily exist.

Children See UCOs Everywhere

For adults, the definition of new foods is simple: these are foods they have never before tasted. However, an unknown food can offer a certain degree of sensory familiarity. That is to say, it can be more or less easily compared to something known. Let us look at some examples illustrating this concept of sensory familiarity.

Let's say I offer you yogurt mousse to taste for the first time. If you are French, like me, this unknown product will nevertheless seem familiar to you to the extent that it is not very different from your usual fare (yogurt and mousse are very common in France). Yogurt mousse resembles what you know: we would say it is a product that presents a high degree of sensory familiarity. Its proximity with the world of the known diminishes the sense of novelty and keeps you from feeling too neophobic at the idea of tasting it.

On the other hand, the first time you were confronted with sushi, a typical Japanese dish, its unfamiliar presentation, texture, and flavor certainly made you feel some distrust. Sushi presents a very low degree of sensory familiarity. It is difficult to compare it to other foods you are familiar with.

From this we can deduce that sensory familiarity, which is the degree of resemblance between an unknown food and the world of the known, modulates neophobia. The less sensory familiarity a food has, the stronger a neophobic response it produces. A food that cannot be compared to something known suffers a loss of identity. It cannot be given a name or even be assigned to a particular category of food.

Children find it harder than adults to compare the unknown to the familiar, for two reasons. The first reason is evident: children have fewer familiar references stored in their memories than adults do. In point of fact, they have experienced much less diversity in foods than their elders have, therefore the links they might establish between the unknown and the known are less numerous. Adults may venture to compare sushi to smoked salmon. Thus, they create for themselves a certain image of sushi, expecting, for example, to experience its texture as slightly slimy. But if smoked fish is unfamiliar to them, children will say that sushi does not remind them of anything, it is totally new, and they do not want to taste it.

Another way of fitting the unknown into the world of the known consists of trying to assign the new product to a familiar group (thus no longer comparing it to one other food in particular). Let us consider the example of the avocado. The fact that it has been assigned to the category of vegetables that are eaten cold allows the French to appropriate it. They know to serve it as an appetizer and dress it with a vinaigrette. Other cultures have classified the avocado as a fruit and thus have appropriated it in some other way.

The concept of classification is not completely mastered before the age of seven. Children only gradually learn to group objects on the basis of common characteristics. And it is all the more difficult if those characteristics are other than physical. For this reason, children learn to recognize a food in one specific form, and not as one among many examples in a group.

Let us consider one last case: soup. Adults know that although form and color vary according to the recipe, all soups have a common denominator. They are liquid preparations of vegetables cooked in water. The concept of soup is assimilated in all its dimensions. However much some specific aspect is altered (color, texture, etc.), everyone understands that it is still a matter of a particular unit within a more general classification.

For young children, soup can be only what they know, and nothing else. As soon as the product is named, they search for the sensory image that is usually associated with it and then form hypotheses on what they are about to taste. The least modification in the presentation or flavor of the food, if it contradicts their hypotheses and runs counter to what they expect, may produce a neophobic reaction.

You can experience this by inviting your child's friend over and asking, "Do you like soup?" The child will answer, "Yes, I often eat soup at home." You prepare soup. But the child makes faces when served, because it is not the soup she knows. For your own child, the inverse will be true. Invited to a friend's house, she will similarly reject the soup made there.

So it seems that because of their more limited experience and their difficulty comparing the unknown to the known, children are often subjected to a whole string of foods that they consider new, rightly or wrongly. Some, they have never tasted. They are unknown, as they would be for adults as well, but they seem less familiar to children because children don't have the capacity to compare them to the world of the known. Others, they have already tasted, but in a different form. In this case, children are not able to connect them to earlier similar experiences.

Thus, the fact that neophobia diminishes with age can perhaps be explained by children's increasingly numerous experiences and their growing capacity to make comparisons and construct categories. Consequently, evolution would appear to be inevitable. Children are induced to taste a constantly growing number of foods, and moreover, they achieve greater cognitive competence. So how can we explain why, even as adults, certain individuals continue to prove neophobic? Is it a matter of a stable personality trait specific to the individual?

Is Neophobia a Personality Trait?

Comparative psychology's objective is, first, to describe the differences between individuals and, second, to explain the reasons for such differences. The comparative approach to neophobia must thus allow us to answer two questions: Are we all neophobic? Why are certain individuals more neophobic than others?

Are We All Neophobic?

If we confine ourselves to the concepts of incorporation anxiety and the omnivore's paradox, the answer to this question would be affirmative: neophobia is a universal trait that characterizes all omnivores. However, the study we have cited by Liliane Hanse shows that children turn out to be more or less neophobic. As cited, 23 percent of children between two and ten years of age are not neophobic and willingly taste any new food without needing any kind of persuasion. On the other hand, we can distinguish three degrees of neophobia among those who are neophobic.

The first degree corresponds to children who ask to taste the dish before deciding whether they are going to eat any more of it. If, on the first mouthful, the food in question does not taste as bad as they might have imagined, they then agree to continue eating it. Thirty-nine percent of children between the ages of two and ten exhibit this first degree of neophobia. It appears that these children demonstrate a certain maturity in their reactions when faced with a new food. Thus, it is not surprising to learn that this group consists largely of children seven years old and older.

The second degree involves children who must be coerced with strong incentives to taste unknown foods. Here we witness certain cases similar to first-degree ones, in which children may continue to eat the food they have been forced to taste, as long as the taste is not as disagreeable as they had expected. This second degree corresponds to about 32 percent of children between the ages of two and ten. These children who adopt a rigid attitude when faced with a new food are, for the most part, between four and six to seven years old.

The third degree manifests a very strong food neophobia. Here, we find children who categorically refuse to taste new foods. Between the ages of two and ten, this applies to about 6 percent of children. Age plays no part here. For some of these children, their neophobia is very clearly outside the norm and does not diminish with age. These children exhibit almost obsessional behavior. The few acceptable foods must always be offered in the same identical form. Problems at the table become intrusive, a cause of concern and repeated conflict. Such children cannot eat away from home. These manifestations are rarely insignificant. They may be the symptom of an underlying, unexpressed anxiety or of difficulty separating from the mother, accompanied by forceful attempts at regression. For a child who exhibits actual phobias in relation to any new food, before any modification in its presentation, a psycho-medical consultation should be considered in order to get a precise and rigorous diagnosis toward the goal of relieving the child's tensions.

Outside of these most difficult cases, we can note changes in attitude running parallel to increasing age. As we have seen, between the ages of four and seven, the majority of children fall, at one time or another, into the second degree. That is to say, they demonstrate very little flexibility in their food choices. They must usually be compelled to taste a new product before they will agree to eat it. Beginning at age seven, the majority of children fall into the first degree. They themselves ask or willingly agree to taste new products. But at any given age, certain children prove to be more neophobic than others.

We do not know how neophobia progresses into adulthood. Whether the most neophobic children become particularly selective adults with regard to food choice is a question that remains to be answered. Still, it is true that we can observe, among adults as well, real differences between individuals. As with children, adults prove more or less neophobic. Most surprising, some adults even prove to be neophilic. These are adults who always seem to be in search of novelty in the food domain. What their shopping carts contain is always different and often includes unfamiliar products that have just come onto the market. At home, their cookbooks are many and varied but principally focus on international cuisine. At restaurants, they will reject trout with butter and lemon for shark fin flavored with cranberries. Finally, when they go abroad, they are eager to taste the local dishes in the countries they visit. Thus, they clearly distinguish themselves from the neophobes, who avoid discovering new gustatory or olfactory sensations and possess a very limited food repertoire, centered around familiar products.

Faced with this individual diversity, a North American researcher, Patricia Pliner, created the food neophobia scale. It involves a ten-item test focusing directly on the relationship between each individual and new foods. It includes statements like "I like to try new foods," "I am afraid of eating foods that I have never tasted before," or "Exotic cuisines seem too strange to me to be eaten." The statements are very simple, and the responses, reported on the scale, are standardized: agree, agree somewhat, disagree somewhat, do not agree at all. What is interesting about the food neophobia scale is that it allows us to predict quite accurately the subjects' actual eating behavior. The most neophobic subjects, according to the scale, do indeed prove more reluctant to taste unknown foods than the more neophilic subjects do.

Pliner created a version of her scale for children. The questions are approximately the same as for the adult scale, but their form is adapted so that parents can respond for their children (for example, "My child is afraid of eating foods he has never tasted before"). Used for children from ages five to eleven, the scale shows that scores do not evolve with age: the scores of five-year-olds are not higher than those of eleven-year-olds. The scale was translated into Swedish and used on a population of fifty-seven families with children between the ages of two and seventeen. The neophobia scores did not evolve between the ages of six and fourteen years. On the other hand, they diminished beginning at fifteen years.

Such results appear to contradict the normal evolution of neophobia with age that was noted in the study by Hanse. This discrepancy can be explained in the light of methodological considerations. In effect, the tools being used to measure neophobia are different in nature. In one case, it is a matter of a scale completed by parents involving general declarations ("My child does not like new foods"); in the other, it is a matter of observed behavior in relation to particular foods ("I noticed that at three years of age my child did not want to try new vegetable X that I offered her"). In fact, Pliner's scale predicts children's behavior less well than adults'. Among children, the neophobia scores correlate only moderately well to their observed willingness to taste any particular new food.

The few studies that have presented children with new products and observed their actual behavior tend to support an evolution in neophobia with age. In studies conducted in 1994 and 1997, Pliner observed that, between the ages of five and twelve, the

DEGREE OF NEOPHOBIA IN CHILDREN (HANSE, 1994)*

Degree of Neophobia†	>2 years, 6 months	2 years, 7 months to 3 years, 11 months	4 years to 5 years, 6 months	5 years, 7 months to 6 years, 11 months	7 years to 8 years, 6 months	8 years, 7 months to 10 years	Total %
0 (eats)	50%	30%	15%	20%	19%	11%	23%
1 (asks)	15%	28%	32%	34%	50%	55%	39%
2 (is forced)	20%	30%	38%	41%	28%	25%	32%
3 (refuses)	10%	8%	11%	3%	2%	5%	6%

* Results of a survey of 579 mothers with children between the ages of two and ten years.
† Each degree of neophobia corresponds to a typical behavior regarding a new food.

older children are, the more adventurous they will be about tasting new foods. In 1995, with a sample of eighty children of four and seven years of age, she observed very precisely that 90 percent of the older subjects were willing to put an unknown product into their mouths (in this case, kasha), as opposed to 35 percent of the younger subjects.

Such an evolution must not disguise the fact that neophilia is always secondary among children. Between the ages of five and twelve, whatever the age, subjects always prefer known foods to foods that are unknown to them. That is not the case among adults. As we have said, some of them prove to be true neophiles. Thus the question remains why, regardless of age, some individuals turn out to be more neophobic than others.

Who Are the Neophobes?

At the present time, no one can answer that question in a convincing and exhaustive manner. Nevertheless, researchers are interested in certain factors that may explain neophobia as an individual characteristic. The first factors they have considered are called identifying factors. They define subjects according to gender, socioprofessional category, and place of habitation.

The gender factor has produced contradictory results. According to the studies, differences may or may not be found in the degree of neophobia among men and women, but the latter in general are perceived as being more reluctant to try new products. This difference has been noted especially in studies on adolescent populations. Young women are generally assumed to be more neophobic than young men. This sends us searching, of course, for other grounds for explanation. What of boys and girls ages two to ten? Are little girls more neophobic than little boys? A study done by Pliner shows, on the contrary, that between the ages of five and eleven girls are slightly less neophobic than boys.

In 1994, Jean-Louis Lambert, a French sociologist, circulated a questionnaire with descriptions of new and traditional food products to 882 adults distributed over different regions of France. The results he obtained showed neophobia to be more common among older people with less education, whereas neophiles were primarily young, affluent urbanites working in upper-level positions and moving in intellectual circles.

Thus, according to this study, the neophobes corresponded mainly to the older, rural sector of the population. These are individuals who reject the idea that new technologies (microwaves) and new places to shop (hypermarkets) or eat (fast-food chains) signify improvements. They show a clear preference for natural, fresh products produced by hand or on the farm.

Nonidentifying characteristics, those traced to the individual personality, have also been considered as explanatory factors for neophobia. In 1997 Pliner conducted a study on adults between the ages of eighteen and seventy-four in which she compared different characteristics specific to each person: their degrees of food neophobia (food neophobia scale) and general neophobia (general neophobia scale); their tendencies to seek out powerful new sensations in four different areas (sensation-seeking scale); the diversity of their experiences in the area of food and their degrees of knowledge about unfamiliar products, such as products coming from foreign countries; their levels of anxiety; and, finally, to what extent they proved to be gourmets.

The results indicated that food neophobia is positively correlated with general neophobia and with anxiety. On the other hand, it is negatively correlated with the pursuit of powerful new sensations and with familiarity with foreign foods. Finally, the fact of being more or less of a gourmet does not correlate with the degree of neophobia.

In other words, neophobes tend to exhibit the following characteristics: they do not appreciate new situations and changes or extraordinary, powerful new impressions, like bungee jumping; they have an anxious temperament; and, finally, they would avoid going to foreign countries or restaurants where they would have to taste unfamiliar products.

Pliner also studied correlations for neophobia among 162 children between the ages of five and eleven. In one stage she evaluated their degree of neophobia, especially by observing their actual behavior when faced with new foods. (In other words, did they choose them from among familiar foods? Did they taste them? Did they like them?) In a second stage she asked their mothers to complete a questionnaire focusing on certain characteristics of their children's temperaments. These characteristics were timidity ("it takes time for my child to warm up to unfamiliar people"); emotionalism ("my child cries easily" or "my child becomes sad easily"); sociability ("my child does not like to play alone" or "my child likes company"); activity ("my child is active immediately upon waking up" or "my child is full of energy").

The scores for neophobia turned out to correlate to two indicators of temperament: the most neophobic children were also the most emotional and the most timid. However, these correlations remained moderate. A very timid or emotional child did not necessarily prove hesitant to taste unknown foods.

Despite this qualification, these results are interesting because they recall a hypothesis already put forward: neophobia is partly the result of a keen sensitivity to tastes and smells. If the most neophobic children are the most sensitive on the emotional and sensory levels, we can conceive of the existence of a center of general sensitivity. Thus, the reaction to taste and to novelty might be one manifestation of a general reactivity, particularly to external stimulation.

But things do not seem so simple, if only for one reason: childhood neophobia essentially centers on the visual aspects of food, and children choose whether to taste a new food or not according to its visual aspect, or its presentation, so that its general appearance allows them to say, "I recognize this" or "I do not recognize this." Thus their decision is based on a purely cognitive criterion. That is why this hypothesis, according to which a high degree of neophobia in a child would be due to a high degree of olfactory or gustatory sensitivity, must be advanced with extreme caution.

Likewise, the other hypothesis according to which the most neophobic children might be in a phase of intense opposition to their parents, though not to be rejected, has yet to be validated at all by experiments.

The last factor considered for explaining individual differences in neophobia is the diversity of previous food experiences. Pliner had subjects eat seven new foods, and then she observed their neophobic tendencies when they were presented with a whole range of unknown products. That is, she counted the number of foods they chose to taste. This number was compared to the neophobic tendencies of another group of subjects who were not preexposed to new foods. The results indicate that people preexposed to novelty prove less neophobic than people who are not.

In order to evaluate the effects of preexposure over a longer term, Capretta undertook an experiment on rats, both immature and adult. He created three drinks of three different flavors unknown to them: vanilla, rum, and walnut. He then formed four groups of rats, each subjected to a specific diet for twelve hours. Three of the groups consumed only one type of drink (vanilla, rum, or walnut), while the fourth group consumed the three types of drinks alternately. At the end of those twelve hours, he offered them a new flavor, a chocolate drink, and observed whether they preferred this new drink or plain water. The results showed that the rats having experienced a diversified diet (vanilla, rum, and walnut) headed more willingly toward the new product than the rats with more limited sensory experiences (vanilla, rum, or walnut exclusively). However, this result was confirmed only among the young rats that had not yet reached maturity.

From these two experiments on the effects of a diverse diet on neophobia, it appears that the more people are exposed to multiple experiences, the less hesitant they are to taste new products. Nevertheless, results obtained from experiments with rats are never directly transposable to humans. We can only venture a claim that an early period of development exists during which the effects of diversity are particularly powerful. In other words, there is no guarantee that offering young children a diversified diet will keep them from becoming neophobic beginning at age two.

Let us note finally that the studies we have been discussing indicate that if neophobia is a personality trait, stable and specific to each individual, its intensity can vary according to the circumstances, for example, the individual's degree of hunger or familiarity with the eating environment.

No research has been able to identify any specific characteristic that reliably predicts whether an individual will be more neophobic or neophilic. What emerges from the various studies is a group of indications that coincide with common sense: older, more conservative, more anxious, and more stay-at-home individuals will be more neophobic. Children who are more sensitive (emotional and reactive to sensory stimulation) will be less adventurous in the area of food. We must understand that neophobia is not just a bad habit but constitutes one of an individual's character traits; it is one manifestation of temperament.

And we must be content for now to recognize food neophobia as a fear, more or less intense according to the individual, that is both universal and normal, especially during childhood. This conception of neophobia as normal, and more or less shared by everyone, ought to permit parents and educators to worry a little less than they sometimes do when faced with sometimes very selective behavior in the children under their charge. But the fact remains that they must search hard for ways to get beyond food neophobia. That is the subject of the next section.

How to Get beyond Neophobia

In concrete terms, how is it possible to get beyond a child's neophobia? How can a food, initially unknown and rejected, become familiar and accepted? The idea is a simple one: the food that is initially rejected must be tasted and retasted many times; as it becomes increasingly more familiar, it is sure to become increasingly more appreciated. In effect, the process of familiarization generally allows for a progressive increase in pleasure. We will first demonstrate this and then attempt to explain it.

The Process of Familiarization

By definition, familiarization involves the passage from the unknown to the known. An object becomes known through exposure to it. For example, you come to know a song through hearing it, a painting through seeing it, a friend through spending time together. Exposure—that is, confrontation with the object or encounters with it—leads to familiarization.

In 1968, the psychologist Robert Zajonc, who works outside the area of food, demonstrated that exposure, and consequently familiarization, allows for greater acceptance of an object. In one of his experiments, for example, Zajonc presented a group of adults with Chinese ideograms that had no meaning to them. He projected the ideograms onto a screen very briefly a certain number of times and then measured, repeatedly, the subjects' preferences for this or that ideogram from a set of several. The adults tended to choose the ideograms that they had previously been exposed to. Zajonc noted that the more often the ideogram was seen, the more easily it was accepted. In other words, known objects were preferred over new objects.

Applications of the idea that we find objects more pleasing as they become more familiar to us, known as "the positive effects of exposure," can be found in our daily lives. That is why a song that might have displeased you when you first heard it finally wins you over as it is frequently played on the radio. Through hearing it, you come to accept it, even to start humming along. This concept is also one of the operating principles behind advertising. The more the image of a certain brand is projected to consumers, the higher the sales for products associated with that brand.

Nevertheless, Zajonc almost immediately encountered detractors, especially Daniel Berlyne, who used experiments to demonstrate the existence of some negative effects of exposure or familiarization. According to Berlyne, novelty prompts curiosity and exploratory kinds of behavior, whereas familiarization leads to lassitude and boredom; in the end, new products are preferred to familiar ones.

From these two contradictory theories, what can we conclude regarding the food domain? Only a few studies have been done. When conducted in a laboratory situation, they usually support the positive effects of exposure. For example, adults may be presented with an unknown food and their degree of acceptance measured. Then they are asked to consume it on a certain number of occasions, spread out over time. At the end of this period of familiarization, their preferences are measured once more. It is generally observed that preference increases following exposure. A food that has become familiar is more appreciated than the same food was when it was unknown, that is, when it was tasted for the first time.

But these studies were done in a laboratory, and we know that the results obtained in experimental contexts are not always directly transposable to the reality of everyday life. When experiments are done in a natural context, we can observe that positive and negative effects of exposure coexist. The positive effects appear over the long term, and the negative ones over the short term. This means that if you present the same food to a subject ten times in a row, he will quickly grow tired of it. But if you intersperse the presentation of this food with other foods, pleasure will increase with exposure.

That is obviously what happens in daily life: we never eat the same food ten times in a row. Good omnivores that we are, our eating repertoire remains quite varied thanks to the combined effects (negative for the short term, positive for the long term) of exposure. Repeated exposure over the long term helps us recognize which foods are good or bad for us, whereas repeated exposure over the short term helps us introduce variety into our diet. Thus, the two effects coexist, and their interaction has an adaptive value for the omnivore, who can gradually diversify his repertoire of consumption in this way.

Nevertheless, the positive effects of exposure on preference over the long term do not occur without fail every time, or at least not without a certain number of exposures. In some experiments, we can observe the neutral effects of exposure—that is, the product tasted twenty times is not more appreciated than the product tasted the first time. It is true that certain conditions can greatly extend the necessary period of familiarization (requiring more than twenty tries).

Some of these conditions involve the characteristics of the tasters: their degree of neophobia, for example. The most neophobic people will be very sensitive to exposure but will need a greater number of exposures than others to accept foods that are initially new. Other conditions involve the foods themselves, especially in terms of their degrees of familiarity and sensory complexity. The least familiar foods and/or the most complex ones on the sensory level risk becoming the objects of lengthy familiarization periods.

The last set of conditions involves the methods of exposure, and especially everything connected to the physical and social contexts for eating. In the presence of neophilic friends, adults will more easily eat foods they would otherwise be reluctant to taste. This is also the case if the environment seems friendly to them or on a special occasion. The neophobe will more easily learn to appreciate sushi when invited out to a Japanese restaurant with friends than when alone at home or with indifferent business associates who might laugh at their hesitations.

Like adults, children are sensitive to this set of conditions. But once more we can observe childhood particularities. To begin, children are more neophobic than their elders as we now know, and thus they need a longer exposure time to accept new foods. Also, when we compare the studies done, we can see that for children certain conditions determine whether or not the positive effects of exposure will appear.

The first is that the food must not be too distasteful initially. If a child exhibits an aversion to a food, a sensory or cognitive distaste, overcoming that initial response will be difficult. No matter how diligent your attempts at gradual familiarization, success will require a long effort. It also seems that in the best-case scenario a food must be eaten at least five times for the positive effects to appear. In other words, neophobia is rarely conquered with the first mouthful.

Thus parents must not admit defeat with their child's first rejection. They must offer the food again from time to time, once a month, for example, without ever giving up. A child three to five years old may, for instance, show a very strong aversion to peas and then learn gradually to accept them until, when she is ten years old, they appear on her list of favorite foods. Parents must respect their children's strong distastes and not force them. However, they also must relinquish the idea that these foods might someday be accepted. Certain aversions do sometimes unexpectedly disappear; your little angel's behavior abruptly changes and he willingly eats a food he formerly detested. But other aversions will last a lifetime.

For children, it is especially important that exposure, or repeated consumption, evolves in a friendly environment where they are not, under any circumstance, ever forced to swallow a food but are, rather, through playful activities offered a taste of it. Children also prove to be responsive to the examples set by their elders. They will more easily agree to try a new product if someone older, an older child or adult, eats it in front of them first.

To summarize, it seems that tasting an initially unknown, unappreciated food many times allows it to become acceptable. That is how adults come to accept the taste of wine, for example. It is gradual familiarization that leads us to appreciate strong sensations we often initially reject, like those produced by alcoholic beverages. As we will see at the end of chapter 5, this is also the principle by which Mexican children become fond of eating the traditional hot, spicy cuisine of their culture. Nevertheless, certain conditions influence whether or not familiarization will have positive effects on preferences. Mexican children are never forced to season their food with hot sauce. It is the friendly environment and the example set by their elders that gradually convert them.

Given the information currently available to us, we cannot predict the amount of time necessary for exposure to produce positive effects. That depends on a kind of alchemy involving the various factors that merge and interact, with the effects produced by one factor sometimes canceling out those produced by another. As a general rule, the stronger the neophobic response, the greater the number of times the food must be tried to become accepted. The more neophobic I am, the more the food displeases me, the more unfamiliar it is to me on a sensory level, the more often I am left alone to try it, or the more often I am with others who strongly influence me—these factors will determine the period of exposure necessary to make me appreciate this food.

Before explaining in detail all the methods for helping children get beyond their neophobia, diversify their diets, and enjoy eating, let us try to understand why, and through what processes, familiarization allows for an increase in preference.

From Familiarization to Pleasure

Three kinds of hypotheses attempt to describe the processes by which food becomes more and more appreciated over the course of familiarization. More or less explicitly and on different levels, all three invoke the role of learning experiences in the gradual acceptance of food. It is a matter of learning experiences that take place over time, through the course of repeated meals. These experiences are nonintentional or, to use a more common term, unconscious. According to the associative hypothesis, the child learns to associate the food with unharmful, even positive, consequences; according to the sensory hypothesis, the child gets used to the taste of the food; and according to the cognitive hypothesis, the child learns to render the food identifiable. Let us try to understand each of these perspectives.

Learning through Association

The associative hypotheses were developed in North America. Paul Rozin and Leann Birch have suggested different hypotheses, but both fall into the category of learning through association. According to this view, people learn—unconsciously and with each eating experience—that a given food is good for them, or at least that it does them no harm. These repeated learning experiences result in a greater acceptance of the food, and in the end it can become the object of a very positive hedonic response.

Rozin proposes what is called the learned safety hypothesis. According to him, familiarization allows for a decrease in incorporation anxiety (which we have already discussed with regard to neophobia in omnivores). Each eating experience that is not followed by toxic effects allows the fear of poisoning to diminish. In turn, this decrease results in a heightening of the pleasure response at the taste of the food. With repeated eating experiences people eventually learn to associate the sensory qualities of the food with its harmless effects on their health.

Birch also focuses on the biological consequences of ingestion, but she proposes that people gradually integrate the positive effects of the food because it relieves their sensations of hunger. According to her, the association between the food's taste and its positive effects occurs on the level of satiation, not on the level of toxicity. The food we unconsciously recognize as having the capacity to satisfy our hunger becomes the one we most appreciate. This could be called the learned satiation hypothesis.

Both the hypotheses of Rozin and Birch rely greatly on the interplay between the sensory qualities of a food (its taste) and its biological qualities (sustaining health, satisfying hunger). Since the food's taste is experienced before the consequences of ingestion, over time the taste becomes the indication of a reassuring ingestive experience. Presented a food that has become familiar, omnivores find the means to calm their anxieties about toxicity and hunger and can eventually take pleasure in tasting what they eat.

Sensorial Experiences and Habituation

Robert Zajonc explains the positive effects of exposure by what he calls the phenomenon of "simple exposure." In fact, he rejects all theories that rely on association. According to him, it is enough for an object to be found repeatedly in a person's perceptive or sensory field (whether seen, heard, touched, smelled, or tasted) for it to become accepted. That is how he explains, for example, that the more often the Chinese ideograms were seen, the more they became the object of a positive hedonic response.

Zajonc's explanation is clear insofar as it rejects associations, but it remains vague to the extent that no other process is proposed. He does not formally explain how familiarization results in heightened pleasure. We must imagine Zajonc's phenomenon of simple exposure as the long-term counterpart to the process referred to as habituation over the short term. Let us consider an example from the olfactory domain.

Surely at some point you have entered a room and been bothered by its stuffy odor. Nevertheless, after a few moments, the odor no longer bothers you. In fact, you no longer notice it. You have gradually become habituated to it. If you leave the room for a certain amount of time and then reenter it, you will once again be surprised by its odor.

We can witness this type of phenomenon over the long term. You no longer perceive the scent of a very familiar person, whereas others, when they meet this person, will not fail to point out what strong perfume she is wearing. With regard to food, progressive exposure to an initially new product may allow us to get used to its sensory qualities to the point that we are no longer disturbed by what seemed surprising to us upon our first encounter.

Cognitive Experiences and Appropriation

The last hypothesis, which Matty Chiva and I both propose, is a cognitive approach that begins with the premise that neophobia is the result of a person's inability to identify a food. He is faced with a UCO (unidentified comestible object), a food that "says nothing to him," according to both meanings of that expression: it is a food that reminds him of nothing he knows, and consequently it offers him nothing he wants. He is going to have to appropriate it—making it a food that is "his"(falling within known parameters) and that pleases him (that is appreciated). Appropriation gradually takes place through successive experiences with the food. Through repeated comparisons between the unknown and the world of the known, he comes to construct an identity for the food, to assign it a familiar meaning.

Now, let us make this hypothesis concrete by offering an example. We had children, ages eight to eleven, taste unknown foods. Then we asked them to describe the foods' sensory qualities by considering their colors, odors, tastes, and textures, but also the foods themselves: "What does this food make you think of? What is it like? What do its color, odor, taste, and texture resemble?"

We then observed that when the food was unknown to them, the children compared it and its sensory qualities to many different images, and they did not appreciate it. One of the foods used over the course of this experiment was dried meat strips, smoked and seasoned. Before tasting it, the children thought the product looked like a chocolate bar. On the other hand, its color seemed close to that of dried fruit, such as dates or prunes. Its odor called up delicatessen products like smoked ham. When the children tasted the dried meat strips, the flavor reminded them of something pungent like hot chili sauce or spices. Finally, they found nothing to which the texture compared, unless it was something inedible, like cardboard, for example.

Subsequently, this product became familiar to them through a series of tastings in natural settings. Over a period of two months the children were asked to eat the strips of dried meat four times, after which they were asked exactly the same questions: "What does this food make you think of? What is it like? What do its color, odor, taste, and texture resemble?" We observed that most of the children succeeded in creating a unified image of the product, which became familiar and the object of a positive hedonic response. The children analyzed the food and its sensory qualities no longer as a series of different images but in a consistent way. The food, including its color, odor, taste, and texture, was generally compared to a delicatessen product, which is how dried meat strips entered the known world. They became familiar because they were consumed a certain number of times, but also because they made their way into the known food repertoire, right beside smoked ham, in the delicatessen category. Eventually the smoked meat strip was no longer an unidentified comestible object but an identified one, able to be appropriated because it fit into known patterns and pleased the children on the hedonic level.

With regard to the various hypotheses we have just presented, no one as yet has offered sufficient experimental verification for associative, sensory, or cognitive learning experiences. Consequently, we cannot say which is the right theory. And it is still an open question as to whether only one or many valid hypotheses exist, because they do not all contradict one another. In effect, food is the source of basic biological changes, multiple sensory experiences, and varied cognitive images. Thus humans have the opportunity to bring food into their domain by appealing to its various properties.

What remains undeniable is this: within the area of food, rejecting novelty most often relates to the fear of a bad sensory experience. In any case, this is part of the reason why children, and even some adults, when asked why they will not eat a new food, reply, "I don't want to taste this food because it isn't good," even though they have never tasted it before. They express their neophobia by centering their discourse on the sensory qualities of the food, and not on their fear of being poisoned, or their feeling of hunger, or their ability to place the food into a known category. Likewise, the food that becomes familiar is appreciated because it is found to be pleasant in the mouth, and not because of its safe, filling, or recognizable nature.

5
Sitting Down to Eat

A sensory image forms in our memory when we taste a food. To this sensory image is attached a hedonic response, either good or bad. That is the reason why we explain our food choices by evoking the taste of the food: I appreciate chocolate for its exceptional flavor; I refuse to eat Swiss chard because of its fibrous texture.

What the omnivore does not know is that this link between the sensory image and the hedonic response is continually strengthened by the metabolic image and information gleaned from the physical and social context. Thus, chocolate may also be appreciated because it is repeatedly offered in a comforting context ("You hurt yourself, here, let me give you some chocolate") or because it is satisfying. Likewise, Swiss chard may be rejected because it is presented in an uncomfortable situation ("Hurry up and eat your vegetables!") or because of once being associated with an upset stomach.

To teach children to appreciate their food, we must keep in

mind that we can simultaneously play on sensory, nutritive, and social aspects.

These are the rules of this game—and I hope you won't find them hard to swallow.

What's for Dinner Tonight?

The question is repeated each day, always the same: what are we eating tonight? Of course, a great number of material contingencies direct our choices: what we have in the refrigerator, how much time we have to prepare the meal, how tired we are. . . . These constraints can be difficult to escape, but beyond that, deciding on a menu should depend on the notions of "good for the health" and "good for the mouth." What we need to find is a balance between these two. And contrary to popular wisdom, they are not always incompatible.

What Foods?

I would like to defend a basic premise. Too many parents ask their children to decide upon their own menus as soon as they learn how to express themselves. It seems to me that it is up to the parents to decide what appears on their children's plates, and not the children themselves. Why? The first reason concerns nutrition. Children cannot know the basic rules of a balanced diet that even as adults we have a hard time mastering. If we let children choose, they will spontaneously go for sweet or fatty foods that satisfy their appetites and give them pleasure. In any case, they will select only foods they already know. Quite obviously, vegetables will rarely appear on the menu.

Of course, one experiment conducted early in the twentieth

century showed that very young children (about one year old) were inherently capable of maintaining a fairly balanced diet over the long term. These young children were observed in an orphanage from the age of six months, and their choices among various foods offered to them were recorded over a period of six to twelve months. At the end of this time, the nutritional quality of their meals was judged satisfactory and their weight acceptable. However, all the foods offered in the study were healthy products. There were no candies, sweetened drinks, or french fries.

The second reason is psychological in nature. Children are asked more and more often and at an increasingly earlier age to demonstrate their autonomy, to make decisions, with the hope, of course, of making them responsible, but also perhaps to show respect for them as individuals. Even if our intentions are good, we must not lose sight of the fact that children are not miniature adults. On the emotional and cognitive levels they must still be protected and given a framework. We do not help our children to grow up by asking them to behave as though they were much older than they are.

Well-known studies in psychology have shown that the best way to help children progress is to situate them just beyond their zone of competence and to guide them in closing the gap between what they know how to do by themselves and what they know how to do with the help of an adult. True respect for children really requires knowledge of their present abilities and adaptation to their rate of development, which will be more or less rapid depending upon the individual.

This is particularly true in the area of food. We have seen that even for an adult having to choose one's food prompts fear and questions concerning the risks involved in eating it. Food choices pose problems for children as well. As evidence of this, let us recall that neophobia begins when children begin to eat all by themselves!

These reasons, nutritional and psychological in nature, lead me to believe that it is preferable to adopt a firm ("this is the menu") and friendly ("that I chose for us") attitude and to encourage your child to taste the dishes represented there. But firmness does not mean rigidity. To be accepted, our adult choices must to some extent take our children's tastes into account. If we decide to have vegetables at least once a day, we must usually choose preferred vegetables and only gradually introduce those that are less appreciated.

Of course, this is a matter of general principle and does not prohibit us from asking children what they would like. If children suggest menus that totally disregard nutrition (french fries, pasta, and chocolate mousse), we can take advantage of the opportunity to discuss the reasons why the chosen menu is inadequate (in simple terms for the very young: too filling, nothing fresh, will not make us strong). And why not take advantage of the opportunity as well to concoct a special holiday meal, horribly inadequate on the nutritional level, but terribly exciting for your child? Like adults, children can understand the notion of the everyday meal, which must consistently provide our necessary nutrition, and the holiday meal. Gradually they can be taught that holidays can also be celebrated without french fries and with more sophisticated dishes.

In the end, this first principle I am proposing requires that we know our children's tastes rather precisely in order to be able to alternate dishes that they select with those they appreciate less. Children are sufficiently affirmative and demonstrative in their preferences that this knowledge is easily acquired, by simple observation of their rejection behavior (pushing away the plate or verbally expressing distaste) or appreciation (empty plate or manifestations of pleasure). Obviously I do not want to encourage here the false notion that children must always be given what they like. That would be absurd. On the other hand, knowing what they like and to what extent they will initially reject something is ultimately a means for trying to accompany them in their explorations of subtle differences and for arousing their curiosity.

This principle also requires that we have an idea of what nutritional balance is. Here, things get complicated. Until our children are two to three years old, the pediatrician or family doctor remains a fairly reliable source of advice (even though medical training remains weak in the area of nutrition). But beyond that age, questions about food are rarely raised with family doctors. Parents find themselves alone in managing the family menu.

Nowadays, the notion of a balanced diet is complex, is subject to many variations, and has been viewed essentially from the perspective of weight control. Excess fat, sweets, and protein alternately find themselves demonized as the cause of weight gain. This approach poses two questions for parents. First, how do we move from nutriments to foods? Second, how do we proceed if a child does not have a recognized weight problem (observed by a doctor)? Given that nutrition is not yet a science that has achieved its final form, it seems judicious to look to the most recent recommendations, repeated frequently in works on balanced diets for children in good health.*

---

*See especially Fricker, Dartois, and du Traysseix, 1998.

1. Require a breakfast that includes a grain product (bread or cereal), a dairy product (milk or yogurt), and fruit (perhaps in the form of juice).
2. Have your child consume at least two raw products a day (vegetables and/or fruit).
3. Offer a cooked vegetable at one or two main meals (lunch or dinner).
4. Remember to favor the consumption of starches (especially bread).
5. Be sure to offer dairy products (yogurt or cheese) at least twice a day.
6. Do not have your child consume meat more than once a day.
7. Restrict consumption of products that are very high in calories (french fries, cold cuts, cake, and so on).
8. Ban sweetened drinks at meals.
9. Restrict snacking on products that are low in nutritional value.
10. Promote exercise (playing a sport or simply walking).

Even though they are very general, these ten recommendations offer the advantage of focusing on foods (not nutriments) and taking into account not just possible excesses (too many products with large amounts of fat or sugar, too much protein) but also possible deficiencies (fiber, vitamins, and minerals). It is a matter of adopting a preventive attitude centered on well-being, rather than a curative approach targeted at the question of weight, which, once again, involves only a limited number of children.

With What Sauce?

The foods chosen to make up the menu are one thing. They must also be cooked and seasoned. Here again I would like to state a fact that bears repeating. At the present time, when we seem more preoccupied with the problem of obesity than the question of taste, it may be healthy to recall that "eating well" has a double meaning: preserving health, of course, but also taking pleasure in eating. Now, contrary to what is generally admitted, the "good grub" that gives us pleasure can also be good for our health.

Let us take an example. Your children never eat the soup that you prepare for them, which is nevertheless a source of invaluable nutrition. But what is this soup? A classic leek-potato recipe to which no cream or milk or Gruyère cheese or croutons may be added? If this recipe suits your children, so much the better. But if not, why deprive them of these ingredients that can add a touch of pleasure to what is simply good for them?

Likewise, spinach can be more or less delectable according to how it is prepared. Its texture, which some people find disagreeable, can be counteracted with the addition of fat. Adding cream offers three advantages. If your child then judges the dish to be good, she will consume it, thus achieving a dose of fibers and vitamins; familiarization with the taste of the vegetable; and a pleasant eating experience. Cream is harmful only if consumed in excess, or if the rest of the meal includes other fatty dishes.

Moreover, the impact of culinary preparation on the rate of food consumption for children is well documented. Observations made by Vincent Boggio of 1,050 meals eaten by French children, ages two to three years, confirm that foods are accepted to varying degrees depending on how they are prepared. In a self-service situation at day care, children had a choice of several appetizers and main dishes. Each day, the staff noted what the children chose, thus providing a precise record of the rate of acceptance of dishes according to their culinary preparation. To offer a few examples:

- Cauliflower, with its specific characteristics that we now recognize, was chosen in 51 percent of the cases when prepared au gratin, in 49 percent when served with a béchamel sauce, in 38 percent when steamed, and in 35 percent in salad.
- Tomatoes: stuffed, 52 percent; in salad, 29 percent; in salad with cucumbers, 28 percent; à la Provençale, 27 percent.
- Leeks: in quiche, 61 percent; with a béchamel sauce, 32 percent; au gratin, 31 percent.
- Green beans: warm, 48 percent; in salad, only 30 percent.

Through these examples we can see that the frequency with which a dish is selected can double according to how it is prepared. Nevertheless, adding something fatty is not the single magic formula for making children eat unappreciated dishes. Let us remember that cooking alters the flavor of the food as well as the texture. Thus, certain foods are preferred warm (green beans) and others cold (tomatoes, carrots). Let us also remember that there are principles of taste some children use when they find themselves faced with new dishes. By increasing the familiarity of an otherwise unknown product, these principles of taste play the role of reassurance. They allow the product to be incorporated at the behavioral level (I will dare to taste it and introduce it into my body) and to be appropriated at the psychological level (I recognize it as my food).

Originally, the principles of taste were shared by members of the same culture. Now we are witnessing a loss of these cultural reference points. Nevertheless, certain individuals systematically embellish their dishes with a familiar seasoning. It may be a matter of a commercial or homemade tomato sauce, mustard, a bit of cheese, or even ketchup.

We maintain that for children without weight problems diagnosed by a doctor, there is no reason to hesitate about adding cream (not in excess) to spinach or butter to green beans.

In What Form?

We have already discussed how the notion of novelty is different for children than for adults. For the child, as many new foods exist as there are ways of presenting any single one.

Accordingly, it is strongly recommended that, at least at first, a food not be prepared in too many different ways. Too great a variety of presentations will risk dissent, conflict, and finally neophobic rejection.

In other words, in order to spark the curiosity that we as researchers and parents are interested in, children need stable, concrete references they are used to. That is particularly true of children between the ages of two and six to seven years, and even more so with neophobic children.

How do we actually set about this? To help a child become familiar with an initially unacceptable soup, we must first establish a reassuring base by always presenting the same preparation, even if it means waiting for the child to mature and become accustomed to the soup. It is only gradually that we can "vary the pleasures" by presenting the soup with new vegetables, or a sprinkle of Gruyère, or a cloud of milk. . . .

It is true that systematic variety in foods is rarely suitable for very young children, who in general prove to be particularly conservative in that area. When it comes to matters of sensory education, it is better to begin with simple, reassuring choices. If your grandmother likes only popular songs and you want to convert her to jazz, it is best to start at the beginning, that is, not to initiate her immediately into the most unrestrained free jazz. As in other domains, food learning experiences are more successful if they take place in a reassuring environment. When too numerous or too violent, they risk leading to withdrawal, rejection, and finally the reinforcement of neophobia.

Hands in the Dough and Words in the Mouth

Of course soup tastes better with a little cream, but the taste of a food is not always enough to make it acceptable. For children, "good" means not only what is prepared well but also what is already familiar to them. Here are two ways of teaching our children to become familiar with what they eat: putting hands in the dough and words in the mouth.

Hands in the Dough

One of the most pleasant and certainly most effective ways of making food familiar is to have children participate in the preparation of meals. Through this contact prior to ingestion, children awaken their senses. They touch and taste in an unconstrained, even playful context. This is the beginning of appropriation, the gaining of knowledge that allows neophobic fear to diminish with regard to what may still be an unknown food. Meal preparation is also a pleasure to do together, to do with and for one another; it is a gift, a kind of miniature "Babette's Feast."

Making contact with raw food can also happen in the garden.

Numerous observations suggest that children are just as stimulated by planting fruits and vegetables and seeing them grow as by cooking the produce themselves. In this regard, of course, young city dwellers are considerably disadvantaged. So why not inspire them to discover the chemistry of "culinary gastronomy"? The chemist and physician Hervé This, who is passionate about cooking, suggests simple recipes for children that reveal molecular secrets, for instance, cheese soufflé, whipped cream, and even boiled water.* This is a matter of food appropriation that is educational and fun (but reserved for children over the age of seven or eight).

All professionals who work with children know this: helping children connect with the products that are used in a dish encourages eating and subsequent pleasure. A study conducted on elementary-school children in outdoor recreation centers offers proof. Based on what remained on the plates, researchers noted that there were fewer scraps when the children had participated in making the meals than when the meals were presented to them all prepared in advance.†

This idea seems to have been assimilated by American parents. In 1989 Paul Rozin did a study in which he asked seventy-six American couples to cite the methods they used to encourage their children to eat vegetables and which they considered to be the most effective. The method most often cited was involving the children in the preparation of meals. But despite being so readily accepted, this idea is rarely put into practice, especially in the present food consumption environment in which a large share of food products are manufactured or prepared in advance.

---

*See This, 1998.
†Unfortunately, for practical reasons schools and day cares tend to have children help make cakes and other pastries. When will they learn to prepare ham with endive in these centers?

That is regrettable. It certainly seems that prepared dishes like frozen foods may offer complete nutrition and positive sensory experiences, but they do not spark children's curiosity about cooking as patiently following a long recipe would. If children help their parents to cook creamed spinach, there is a better chance they will eat it than if they simply watch their parents stick a container in the microwave. On another level, for example with very young children, rather than suggest they go choose a fruit-flavored yogurt from the refrigerator, we can spark their curiosity by giving them plain yogurt and asking them to add their choice of available ingredients: jam, cereal, pieces of fresh fruit, and so on.

This is, of course, a case against overreliance on ready-to-eat foods. Despite their practical aspects, we must know how to resist the regular use of prepared products that strike children, who lack any other information or experience, as objects coming from nowhere, void of all significance. To put children's hands in the dough is to make their mouths water. And as we are about to see, it is also a way to oil their tongues.

Words in the Mouth

"Sensory education" is a term used more and more often since Jacques Puisais created "taste classes."* These consist of ten training sessions, each an hour and a half long, conducted in French primary schools. During these sessions, the children, while making

---

*See Puisais and Pierre, 1987.

unfamiliar dishes, are invited to discover tastes and the words to express them.

The idea behind sensory education is to find ways to go beyond the initial hedonic response of all individuals in relation to food, that poor dichotomy of "this is good" or "this is not good." This response is spontaneously expressed in the first place because it has a biological value for the individual to the extent that it directs behavior: if I like it, I will eat it; if not, I will leave it on my plate.

Applying words to our foods, to the sensations they produce, can help children get beyond this simplistic hedonic response. Words have the virtue of calming the omnivore's anxiety. They are learned within a cultural system in situations involving social interaction and thus serve as a springboard to the world of the known and the reassuring. Constructing a verbal image of a food is a way of transferring it from the stage of unidentified comestible objects to the stage of identified comestible objects. Naming gives meaning to those external objects that we must put inside us. Children who know what they are going to eat are thus prepared for the sensory experience they are going to have and so adopt a less neophobic, more nuanced attitude.

Children can be educated on the sensory level in the same way they can be taught to appreciate music or to discover any art or sport: through gradual sensitization. But it is a delicate operation on two accounts. First, food is the thing that offers the most complex sensory bouquet. Let us recall that the eyes, hands, nose, tongue, trigeminal nerve, ear, and jaw—thus involving sight, touch, smell, and then taste, smell for a second time, the sixth sense, hearing, and then touch once again—all participate in the appreciation of food. Tasting is thus, simultaneously, seeing, touching, feeling, smelling, tasting, hearing, chewing, and swallowing (see chapter 1). Second, as adults we ourselves lack vocabulary in the olfactory and gustatory domains. Much as children do, we spend a lot of time eating, though without taking the time to discuss the contents of our plates.

So we must begin at the beginning: to name for children the dish being offered to them. And why not announce it dramatically, like a waiter at a fine restaurant? "Presenting our mashed potatoes and roast pork!" Why not mention the secret recipe; the appearance, color, and form; or the memories the dish conjures? Then, we need to embark upon a more analytical campaign, working from sense to sense. First, we can focus on the texture to the touch and the scent to the nose, preparing the child for the sensations to be discovered by tasting the dish. Once it is introduced to the mouth, we can evoke its flavor, especially its olfactory and gustatory qualities.

With regard to texture, it is easy to teach children to distinguish "hard" from "soft," as these two contrasting terms belong to their general vocabulary. Beginning there, we must articulate the nuances: "soft" declines into delicate, smooth, chewy, gummy, sticky; "hard," into firm, crisp, crusty, coarse. . . . We must also get children into the habit of choosing fruit from the basket according to its ripeness, testing the freshness of bread by squeezing it, or assessing the crunchiness of cereals by crumbling them. Finally, the "noise game" appeals particularly to younger children. Offer children a new food to taste and ask them to predict the sounds it will make when they chew it. Once aroused, their curiosity will help them taste the food.

With regard to smells, learning takes on a different character. Let us recall that to penetrate the domain of odors is to discover a universe both enormously rich and virtually unknown to scientists. Although the physiologies of sight and sound are well known, the workings of our olfactory system remain largely unexplored.*

With no objective scientific data available, it has never been possible to establish a satisfactory classification of odors, as exists for colors, for example. In effect, each shade can be assigned to a specific abstract category, like blue, red, or yellow.

Olfactory categories do not exist; the denomination of odors is thus made by analogy, that is, in reference to known objects that have a concrete existence. That amounts to saying that the most satisfactory way of describing the odor of a food is giving the food's name. We can speak of the odor of strawberries only by saying, "That smells like strawberries." Although we can, of course, add that it smells "like fruit" or "fresh," we must still return to the very source from which the smell emanates.

Furthermore, unlike the four terms that illustrate tastes with which we must be satisfied, there exist a very great number of olfactory descriptors. Specialists, trained to describe smells as singers are trained to follow musical scores, can describe with complete precision up to fifteen thousand odors. Our normal language includes three or four hundred terms for them. This system, simultaneously limited and rich, makes olfactory sensory education difficult. It would be a shame to renounce it. And there is often a mutual pleasure in sensitizing children to different odors by teaching them to smell foods and give names to what they perceive.

---

*First, we do not know what in the olfactory molecule is responsible for the odors we experience; there is no case in which its observation under a microscope allows us to predict its odor. Moreover, we have discerned that two very closely related molecules can produce totally different sensations in the nose and in the mouth. Second, we are just as ignorant about the processes by which our receptor cells perceive those odors.

Developing this habit offers two advantages. First, children become aware of the fact that odors for the nose are also perceived in the mouth. Smelling food thus prepares them for the mouth's sensory experience. Second, through olfactory sensations they discover new foods in trying to compare them to known foods. To the extent that odors are named by analogy, identifying them consists of comparing them to the odors of familiar foods. Children will try to compare the odor of a new fruit to that of other fruits that belong to their known repertoire. This is a way of familiarizing themselves with the food. It may seem a little tentative, but to my knowledge we have no better pedagogical system at the moment.

Considering the ambiguities that we have raised, learning to name tastes is both simple and complicated. It is simple because only four gustatory descriptors exist: the sacrosanct sweet, salty, sour, and bitter. It is complicated because two of these terms, sour and bitter, are the subject of widespread semantic confusion. We qualify as bitter the taste of cabbage, zucchini, endive, grapefruit, dark chocolate, coffee, and beer. However, among these various products no common chemical denominator has been identified. On the other hand, it seems obvious that this expression refers to a disagreeable sensation, especially for children.

The same is true for sour, for which the chemistry is better understood. Children tend to use the expressions "that's sour," "that's strong," "that's sharp," "that's hot," and even "that's bitter" and "I don't like that" indiscriminately. On a daily basis, and through successive attempts, we can teach them to distinguish these various expressions.

For sweet and salty, children can make easy reference to the crystallized products we use in cooking. A simple experiment consists of having a child taste plain yogurt and then yogurt with a pinch of sugar added, with each spoonful having another pinch added. The child should subjectively judge the intensity of the perception: is there too little or, on the contrary, too much sugar? The same procedure can be followed adding salt to a bowl of soup.

Finally, we must counter the habit of believing that each product corresponds to a single taste. In talking about food, it is clear that we must use not just one of the four landmarks (sweet, salty, sour, or bitter) but more often at least two of them. Lacking other means, we can always find nuances in these four dimensions, get to know each one better, and learn to combine them.

Sensory education requires some modicum of availability on the part of adults and children, and in this regard it cannot be practiced every day, no matter what the circumstances. However, this learning can be presented as a playful way to have children taste foods. Children are great experimenters and will eagerly agree to participate in the game of sensory discovery. The rules for it are easy. Very young children should be addressed in simple language: "Here is the food. Do you think it is going to be crunchy? Will it make noise when you chew it? Can you tell me what it reminds you of when you taste it? What is it like in your mouth?" Then you name and describe the food with the child. As Jacques Puisais put it so well, we must let the foods tell their story, and we must teach children to play the whole sensory field. By developing their senses, we can wager on seeing them gradually refine their judgments and one day pass from the stage of gourmand to gourmet.

Warning: Sensory Education Is Not Nutritional Education

Nutritional education programs focus essentially on a healthy diet. They are generally a matter of programs offered in schools in which children are taught to recognize the different categories of foods (which contain fat, calcium, protein, fiber, and so on), as well as good food habits that benefit health and bad food habits to be avoided.

Certainly children must be informed about food's essential role in helping their bodies to function well. Adults are capable of understanding the long-term benefits of certain foods in the body. They have an idea of the reasons for consuming vegetables and the effects of calcium, and they know it is best to avoid fatty foods, which can cause cardiovascular diseases in humans. These are arguments that children have a hard time integrating, not because they are not interested in them, but because they do not have the cognitive capacity to assimilate these phenomena.

Many experiments have demonstrated this. Until the ages of ten to twelve, children do not understand the principles according to which ingested foods function to build the body over the long term. According to Jean Piaget's theory, until this age children are in the stage of so-called concrete operations. They can reason only about objects that they can manipulate. Nutriments remain a totally abstract idea for them; they do not truly assimilate this type of knowledge.

At the present time, nutritional education, with its focus on diet, tends to override sensory education on the grounds that there are more and more obese children. Americans seem to be totally obsessed with aspects of health, to the detriment of sensory concerns, yet nevertheless the United States sees its obesity numbers growing day by day. France, in contrast, long famous for its culinary sensibilities, has developed a different culinary culture.* One experiment demonstrates this. Presented with three foods—pasta, bread, and sauce—American adults were asked to link two of them. Then French adults were asked to do the same. In most cases Americans thought about the nutritional aspects; thus they linked the carbohydrates—that is, the pasta and bread. The French, on the other hand, thinking in terms of taste, linked either the sauce with the pasta or the bread with the sauce.

Another study along the same lines was conducted by Pliner in 1995. She asked eighty children, ages three to eight years, to taste new foods. To half the children she said, "Taste this, it's good for you." To the other half she said, "Taste this, it tastes good." In most of the cases she observed, only the information "It tastes good," and not "It's good for you," allowed children to overcome their initial neophobia. This obviously argues for a sensory education for children, and not a nutritional one, which is of more interest to adults.

At home, it is better to choose the family menu taking into account a balanced diet and avoiding a focus on the question of weight for children (and especially for girls). Because it can produce guilt, the question of weight is capable of disturbing the relationship with pleasure that we are all entitled to maintain with our food.

---

*Let us note that obesity affects only a small minority of the French population, although its incidence is rapidly increasing.

Don't Finish
What's on Your Plate

Here is a phrase, inherited from a past still sensitive to food short-ages, that rings a familiar bell: "Finish what's on your plate." I would like to offer three arguments suggesting that routinely urg-ing children to clean their plates can interfere with their ability to regulate their appetites. Of course, hunger and satiation are pri-marily biological signals that do not need to be learned. But as we will see, they can be altered by experience.

The Effect of Sensory Satiation

If I offer you a sample of a strong-tasting cheese, its sensory quali-ties will lose their intensity with just a few mouthfuls, after which you will no longer perceive its flavor. I am in the process of eating my soup; on the third spoonful, I feel the need to add salt, pepper, and cheese to give my soup more taste. These signs are the conse-quence of the effects of sensory satiation.

This kind of satiation is qualified as sensory because it occurs in relationship to the taste of the food (its flavor). American researcher Barbara Rolls first demonstrated that we very quickly get used to the flavor of a food. The sensations that a food pro-duces in us diminish quite rapidly over the course of a meal. The receptor cells adapt, reacting less strongly with repeated stimula-tion, in the same way that our noses get used to the odor of a room after we have been in it for only a few moments.

That is why it is common to observe eaters seasoning their dishes after a few mouthfuls. We grind pepper over our salads, squeeze lemon on our fish, add hot sauce to our couscous, pour raspberry sauce over our cottage cheese, and so on. This behavior conveys our pursuit of gustatory, olfactory, and trigeminal sensations, which come to compensate for the loss of sensations produced by the food itself.

The effect of sensory satiation has the functional and adaptive value of prompting us to consume another food in order to quickly restore flavor in the mouth: We seek out a food that offers a very different flavor than what we have just tasted. That is the reason why both children and adults eat more if they have ten different dishes to consume than if they are served an appetizer, an entrée, and a dessert. With each new food, their appetite is reawakened. For those who want to eat less, this kind of unconscious incentive to consume can be an inconvenience, but for those who want to adapt and, as good omnivores, vary their menus—that is to say, for the species in general—it is an advantage.

In the light of Rolls's work, we can understand the attitude of children who refuse to finish their dinners but happily agree to eat their desserts as something other than trickery ("I'm not hungry for my creamed celery anymore"). This is how children signal that the dish no longer stimulates their senses. Nevertheless, dessert, with its very different gustatory and olfactory characteristics, will be the source of renewed pleasure.

Caloric Compensation: Wisdom of the Body

The human machine is programmed to eat when it is hungry and to stop consuming when it has attained a certain state of repletion. The body seems to have the innate wisdom to eat to survive, that is, to relieve its sensations of hunger. It seems that children know better than adults how to regulate consumption according to the biological signals of hunger and repletion. What adults consume over the course of a meal depends little on what they consumed for appetizers. Their appetites are stimulated by what their plates contain (external information), independent of their degree of hunger (internal information). On the other hand, the amount of food ingested at the table by children seems adjusted to their earlier consumption of appetizers.

However, children allocate their meals quite variably from one day to the next. They exhibit the peculiarity of consuming very different amounts of calories from one meal to the next. This trait has interested researchers. In the early 1990s Leann Birch, for example, observed the meals taken by fifteen children, ages two to five years, for six days. Taking into account the day's meals (breakfast, lunch, snack, and dinner) and also between-meal nibbling in the morning and evening, Birch measured the number of calories ingested each time.*

The results showed that from one day to the next the variations were insignificant—on the order of 10 percent—while, as is often true in the area of food, individual differences remained very noticeable. But the great majority of children, day by day, exhibited very significant variations from one meal to the next. That may simply mean that they were adjusting one meal based on another. If they had a big lunch, they would have a smaller snack. And if they had a smaller snack, they would eat more at dinner. We must respect this natural adjustment and, in order to do so, not urge children to routinely finish everything on their plates.

In alignment here with purely dietary considerations, we can thus affirm that it is better for children to consume the greatest amounts over the course of their regular meals; this helps to avoid,

---

*The term "nibbling" is not, to my mind, a pejorative, since it is true that young children need to eat more often than adults.

especially in the case of older children, a very significant intake at snack time of products that are low in nutritional value.

Although children in general have the ability to adjust their food intake, great differences among individuals exist in this area, a topic we will turn to presently in reference to so-called internal and external subjects.

The Internals and the Externals

We say that individuals have strong internality standards if they easily recognize the biological signals emitted by their bodies. In other words, such people adapt themselves very well to their hunger and repletion, initiating their meals when they are hungry and ceasing to eat when they are full. On the other hand, other people exhibit strong externality standards. The quantities they ingest are largely conditioned by external signals regarding meals: social pressures ("Let's eat!"), cultural pressures (the habitual mealtime), or the contents of their plate. If they have before them foods they appreciate, they do not hesitate to continue to consume them, even if they have no longer been hungry for the past fifteen minutes. These are the people who always clean their plates and never refuse dessert, even after a hearty meal.

This individual characteristic surfaces more or less strongly depending on the time of day and the particular meal. Even though "internal" and "external" individuals cannot be listed according to a particular typology, it has long been believed that obesity may be the result of strong externality standards. In 1994 Birch conducted a study to examine this issue. She measured the caloric adjustment ability of seventy-seven children, ages two to four years, some of whom were significantly overweight. She did not find a notable link between the "adjustment" and the "overweight" variables.

However, the heaviest children were the ones who exhibited the least capacity to adjust (in this study, the girls on average performed less well than the boys).

Birch also evaluated the feeding style of the mothers and assessed its effect on caloric adjustment ability. It appeared that the mothers who exerted the most control over food intake (requiring that food be eaten only at meals rather than in response to a sensation of hunger, requiring that everything on the plate be eaten) had children with the least sensitivity to the caloric values of foods.

From this ingenious study we could draw the conclusion that excessive parental control leads to a drop in the caloric adjustment ability of children, and consequently to weight problems. But first, these results merit confirmation through more numerous studies. And second, we know there is a strong hereditary component to obesity.

Still, parents may be advised to stop insisting that children absolutely finish everything on their plates. That is not to say that children must be allowed to adjust entirely on their own, under the pretext that they are fully capable of adapting to the biological signals they perceive. But when children have already eaten half their green beans or their pasta, they must have the freedom to say, "I am stopping; I'm not hungry anymore." The epoch in which children were required to clean their plates so as not to waste food is long past.

In reality, the main thing is to remain vigilant. We do not need to force children to clean their plates if they are really no longer hungry or if they seem put off by the food before them, but we can also watch to see that this is not a pretext used repeatedly for not finishing what they do not want to eat and then possibly making up for it at dessert time.

Children must be taught to remain sensitive to their sensations of hunger and repletion, thus reinforcing their internality rather than their externality standards. Let us consider two examples. A child who wants to have candy for a snack will say, "I'm hungry. Can I have some candy?" Without refusing this request, you can answer, "Are you hungry or do you want to eat candy?" In this way she quickly learns the difference between the two terms.

It is also necessary to get into the habit of serving children small quantities. If a child asks for a second helping, ask him whether he is still hungry ("Is there room in your stomach?") before automatically complying with his request.

Finally, let us recall that exposure allows for familiarization with the taste of a food. While we needn't require children to finish what is on their plates, we can still encourage them to taste what is being offered.

Let's Eat, Everyone!

The pleasure center simultaneously assimilates sensory information and all other information drawn from the consumption context. I am going to discuss some experiments that demonstrate precisely the effect of the social and emotional context on the establishment of food preferences.

Give Them a Model

Children rarely eat alone. When consuming food, they are always in the company of adults or even other children. We must try to understand the effects of such company on the development of preferences and aversions. As early as 1938, a researcher by the name of Karl Duncker demonstrated that telling stories in which the hero likes a food not yet appreciated by children tends to increase their receptivity toward it. The best example is still Popeye and his famous spinach.

More recently, in 1975, Harper and Sanders devised an experiment comparing the role of the mother to that of strangers with regard to the acceptance of new foods. The reactions of eighty children (forty two-year-olds and forty four-year-olds) were observed when alternately their mother and a researcher unknown to them proposed a new food. In this case it was an omelet with ham, blue cheese, and macadamia nuts. Half the mothers proposed the food by means of a simple offer: they asked their children to taste it. The other half tasted the food before asking their children to taste it (a situation of preliminary tasting). The unknown researcher did the same, approaching half the children with a simple offer and the other half with a preliminary tasting.

The results indicate that when the adult tasted the food before offering it, 80 percent of the children agreed to eat it, as opposed to 47 percent when the food was simply offered. Moreover, when the food was offered without being tasted, the mothers had more success in getting the children to taste it than the researchers did. The discrepancy between the success of the mothers and that of the researchers was greater still for the younger children when the adults tasted the food.*

Thus, it appears that through simple observation very young children manage to control their neophobic tendency. Patricia Pliner obtained similar results among adults. Even neophobic

---

*We will recall the similar situation of young rats who, when induced to taste unknown foods, also waited until their parents or adult rats had tasted those foods before doing so themselves.

subjects more easily agreed to taste a new food if another subject tasted it preliminarily in front of them.

As for Birch, she conducted an experiment on the influence of peers in establishing food preferences among preschool-age children (ages three to five years). First, she measured the appreciation of forty children in a solitary situation for nine different vegetables. Then she arranged the children around a dining-hall table according to those preferences. The "target" child, who preferred vegetable A to vegetable B, was seated with three or four other children who exhibited the reverse preference (vegetable B to vegetable A).

These two vegetables were served over the course of four meals, and the children had to choose between them at each meal, with the target children choosing last. Among the fifteen target children who chose their preferred food at the first meal, ten were observed opting for the other food at the fourth meal. The rates of consumption corroborated those obtained for the choices: as the days passed, the amounts of the unappreciated food that were consumed grew for the target children, whereas they remained the same for the others.

Finally, the children were once again observed privately to evaluate the evolution of their appreciation for the two products, without the presence of their peers. It appeared that the initially less-liked vegetable was significantly better appreciated by 82 percent of the subjects (fourteen out of seventeen). Conversely, the initially preferred vegetable was less appreciated by 71 percent of them (twelve out of seventeen). The results of these experiments indicate that, here again, children proceed by observation. Seeing peers accept, appreciate, and consume a product they do not appreciate themselves, they modify their food behavior by adopting that of their peers—and this is true even when their peers are no longer present. It is not simply "monkey see, monkey do"; the preference has truly become internalized.

Such data clearly shows that, through exposure to a model set by others, food acceptance can be modified by social learning. Thus, a neophobic subject will be reassured by witnessing the new food being consumed by familiar individuals. The effects of exposure are even more dramatic if children consume the food in the company of individuals they see taking pleasure in tasting it. Among young children, parents or familiar adults very clearly offer the most powerful models, whereas older children will be more strongly influenced by the presence of their peers. Nevertheless, though children learn as they grow up to differentiate themselves from their parents, their parents long remain models to whom they refer and who are capable of modifying their tastes.

Give Them Love

Birch wanted to demonstrate how the emotional tone of the consumption context influenced children's appropriation of food. In this experimental design, she asked sixty-four children, three to five years of age, to taste eight little sweet or salty sandwiches and to offer a hedonic appreciation of each: I do not like it, I am indifferent, I like it. For each child she selected the sandwich that was his or her median preference and offered it to that child just once a day intermittently over a period of six weeks, for a total of twenty-four times. The children were divided into three groups, each consuming the food in a particular context.

In the first context, which we can call the nonsocial context, every day the children were told, "Remember that you have your little sandwich waiting for you in your cubby, and if you're hungry you can go eat it." The second context was a warm, social context in which an adult stayed with the children while they ate their sandwiches at some random time in the day. The third context involved a social reward, in which children were presented their sandwiches contingent upon doing something good like answering a question well in school, behaving well, or playing well with other children. They were specifically told that they were being given their sandwiches as a reward.

The evolution of the children's preferences was measured at the end of four weeks, again at the end of six weeks, and a final time six weeks after the experiment ended. For food consumed in the nonsocial context, the results indicated that no evolution of preference was observed (the effects of exposure being nullified). The child did not learn to accept the food.

On the other hand, in a warm, friendly context, whether or not with the reward contingency, and even after a six-week interval, the preference for the food grew in an altogether significant way, and even more significantly for the food consumed as a reward. In other words, children tend to associate the taste of a food and the warm, friendly context in which it is consumed, which confirms what we know about how the pleasure center functions. The warm context adds to the hedonic value of the product. For this reason, it is in our interest to present new foods only if we feel we are sufficiently available to create an agreeable atmosphere.

For ethical reasons, the study was not extended to observe the effects of a negative socioemotional context on the evolution of preferences. However, we could imagine that, in the opposite way, tumultuous and constraining contexts would create a rejection associated with the taste of the food. This implies that ideally we must show ourselves to be constantly available, open and ready to calmly handle conflicts. This is, of course, the ideal. . . .

Give Them Spinach as a Reward

The experiment we have just described showed that using food as a reward promotes its appreciation. Another experiment was done in which foods were used not as rewards, as an end goal in themselves, but as a means, in a purely instrumental fashion. Children were invited to drink an unknown fruit juice in order to receive permission to participate in some fun activity, such as playing outside or watching a movie. The results indicated that for nine out of twelve children, the preference for the juice consumed in this instrumental fashion diminished after the phase of familiarization.

If we are to believe the children, it is generally true that anything used as a means tends to diminish or depreciate in its acceptance. It is as if these young minds say to themselves, "If I'm rewarded for accepting this, then it must be bad. . . ."

This comparison between food-as-reward and food-as-means clearly seems to contradict the validity of our most common practices. When children cry, are hurt, or are sad, to console them we give them candy. Thus, we tend to increase the acceptance of a sweet product, which, in general, we do not want to do. Conversely, when we want to make them accept spinach, about which they grumble, we tell them to eat their spinach so they can have dessert and leave the table. This tends to diminish the acceptance of the vegetable—exactly the opposite of the intended goal.

Of course, that does not mean that we should never offer children candy or never tell them to finish their spinach before leaving the table. It simply means that parents must be aware of the outcome of this kind of education method. No hypothesis suggests that using vegetables as a means will make them more easily accepted. But we should avoid the "if you don't finish your spinach, you won't get dessert" line and sometimes try to console our children with treats that are healthier than candy (an apple to crunch, a carrot to nibble).

A True Story to Digest

Observations made in Mexico by the indefatigable Rozin show how exposure, example, and context contribute to the development of preferences, even to the point of reversing a natural tendency: the rejection of hot peppers.

Rozin made himself welcome in the homes of Mexican families in order to observe their behavior at meals, and especially to see how hot peppers were presented. He wanted to learn how children, between the ages of one and ten, come to lose their ability to pass up hot pepper, which is initially rejected since it produces a burning sensation.

He noted that beginning when children are two years old, hot sauce is set on the table, and parents invite the children to help themselves to this seasoning when eating enchiladas, for instance, to put the right finish on their traditional meals; but they are not compelled to do so. For the older children, eight years and above, enchiladas are served with hot sauce. In effect, as observed between two and eight years of age, children gradually come to supplement their foods with this sauce by themselves, through observing its use and with no pressure from the adults. Between the ages of two and three, they hardly use this sauce at all. Beginning at three years, they dip the end of their enchiladas into it. Certainly by five years of age, they feel the need to supplement their dishes with it. Deprived of the seasoning when offered the same menu, these children were completely lost; they clamored for hot sauce in order to eat their meal.

All we need to do is proceed similarly with vegetables in our own cultural repertoire. . . .

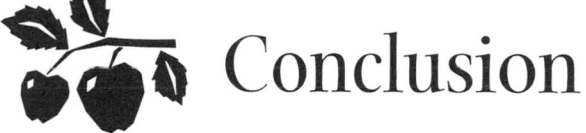 Conclusion

As you have seen, the development of taste is such a complex business that I have given up on the idea of writing a book of ready-to-use psychological recipes. Contrary to what certain psychologists would have us think, there exists no single educational model that is valid for all parents and children. Education comes through knowledge and cannot consist of following some guide to good behavior without understanding the basics.

That is why I have made it my objective to inform you about the ingredients of a potential taste education. It is up to each one of us to assimilate this sometimes indigestible knowledge and to get our children to try the sauce, each according to our own means. Mine are limited: My temperament is, by nature, impatient, and I am no great cook, nor even an exceptional taster. I did not have the wisdom to raise my children with a man much more available or organized than I am.

And nevertheless our sauce is well received. Our daughters feast on cauliflower, spinach, and other green vegetables, appreciate the strong flavor of a Muenster or Boursin cheese, and can recognize different fruits by scent with their eyes closed. "It is a real pleasure to have them at the table," as their grandmother would say. My work as a researcher and my penchant for pleasure have guided me considerably throughout this learning experience.

But these two ingredients may not be enough. How can I explain, for example, my daughters' immoderate taste for cauliflower? Is it because they are nontasters of PTC? Is it because their grandmother cooks this vegetable wonderfully and she appreciates the help of her little kitchen crew? Because I taught them to compare the crunchiness of the raw vegetable to the way it melts when cooked? Because I did not give up serving it to them after their initial rejections? Because I appreciate it myself, which keeps me from modeling to them contagious grimaces of disgust when we sit down together at the table to calmly discuss our day (leaving out the bad grades)? So many factors can play a part in the education of taste!

Rest assured, however, that my daughters remain children who, like others, leap on the candy offered at birthday parties, enjoy adding ketchup to their pasta, and eagerly choose chocolate mousse over a peach for dessert. Above all, they remain distinct from each other, and that is sometimes the most disconcerting thing. One of them is quite simply neophilic. Though sweet products are her cup of tea, she will willingly taste any new food offered to her. The other one proves more difficult and, despite my continual efforts, refuses to eat peas, kidney beans, and lentils, for example. She now knows to answer me with "Even if others like them, for me they're disgusting!" and "No, I'm not being difficult, though maybe hypergeusic" (that sounds so much more chic). But

I can see her growing up; she is becoming more and more open to novelty . . . and a very fine taster.

What I know about taste (and what I hope you have now appropriated) has helped me to understand my daughters' reactions, development, and differences. Nevertheless, understanding does not mean completely accepting. I know how to say no. I also know how to say yes. When, for example, I invite them to taste a new dish, I think it gently teaches them the pleasure of discovery, of being open and sharing. Perhaps, in writing this book, that is what I have hoped to do with you. It is another big wager, but so rewarding!

Bibliography

I used many scientific works and articles to write this book. Attaining them someti mes proves difficult for the general public. Thus, I have made a choice; the only references I cite here are French works available in all good bookstores.

Apfelbaum, M., ed. *Risques et peurs alimentaires* [Food Risks and Fears]. Odile Jacob, 1998.

Bonnet, C., and J. Hosselopp, eds. *Des goûts et des odeurs* [Tastes and Odors]. Psychologie Française, no. 41/3. Dunod, 1996.

Bruner, J. S. *Car la culture donne forme à l'esprit* [For Culture Gives Form to Spirit]. Eshel, 1991.

Chiva, M. *Le doux et l'amer* [The Sweet and the Bitter]. PUF, 1985.

Corbin, A. *Le miasme et la jonquille* [The Miasma and the Daffodil]. Flammarion, 1982–86.

Dulau, R., and J.-R. Pitte, eds. *Géographie des odeurs* [A Geography of Odors]. L'Harmattan, 1997.

Fischler, C. *L'homnivore* [The Omnivore]. Odile Jacob, 1990.

Flandrin, J.-L., and M. Montanari. *Histoire de l'alimentation* [A History of Food]. Fayard, 1996.

Fricker, J., A.-M. Dartois, and M. du Fraysseix. *Guide de l'alimentation de l'enfant—De la conception à l'adolescence* [A Guide to Feeding Children: From Conception to Adolescence]. Odile Jacob, 1998.

Giachetti, I., ed. *Identité des mangeurs, image des aliments* [The Identity of Eaters, the Image of Foods]. Polytechnica, 1996.

———, ed. *Plaisir et préférences alimentaires* [Pleasure and Food Preferences]. Polytechnica, 1992.

Herbinet, E., and M. C. Busnel, eds. *L'aube des sens* [The Dawn of the Senses]. Les cahiers du nouveau-né, no. 5. Stock, 1991.

Lambert, J.-L. *L'évolution des modes de consommation alimentaire en France* [The Evolution of Food Consumption Styles in France]. Lavoisier, 1987.

Lévi-Strauss, C. *Le cru et le cuit* [The Crude and the Cooked]. Plon, 1965.

Pfirsch, J.-V. *La saveur des sociétés: Sociologie des goûts alimentaires en France et en Allemagne* [The Flavor of Societies: A Sociology of Food Tastes in France and Germany]. Presses Universitaires de Rennes, 1997.

Puisais, J., and C. Pierre. *Le goût et l'enfant* [Taste and Children]. Flammarion, 1987.

Rufo, M., ed. *Bébé à l'huile, bébé au beurre* [Baby in Oil, Baby in Butter]. Erès, spirale no. 4, 1997.

Schaal, B., ed. *L'odorat chez l'enfant: perspectives croisées* [The Sense of Smell in Children: Crossed Perspectives]. Revue Enfance, no. 1/97. PUF, 1997.

This, H. *La casserole des enfants* [The Children's Casserole]. Belin, 1998.

Editions Autrement,
Mutations/Mangeurs Series:

Blanc-Mouchet, J., ed. *Odeurs: L'essence d'un sens* [Odors: The Essence of a Sense]. No. 92, 1987.

Piault, F., ed. *Nourritures: Plaisir et angoisse de la fourchette* [Foods: Pleasure and Anguish from the Fork]. No. 108, 1989.

Danziger, C., ed. *Nourritures d'enfance: Souvenirs aigres-doux* [The Foods of Childhood: Bittersweet Memories]. No. 129, 1992.

Piault, F., ed. *Le mangeur: Menus, mots et maux* [The Eater: Wares, Words, and Wrongs]. No. 138, 1993.

N'Diaye, C., ed. *La gourmandise: Délices d'un péché* [Gluttony: A Delectable Sin]. No. 140, 1993.

Fischler, C., ed. *Manger magique: Aliments sorciers, croyances comestibles* [Magical Eating: Sorcerous Edibles, Edible Beliefs]. No. 149, 1994.

Bessis, S., ed. *Mille et une bouches: Cuisines et identités culturelles* [A Thousand and One Mouths: Cultural Cuisines and Identities]. No. 154, 1995.

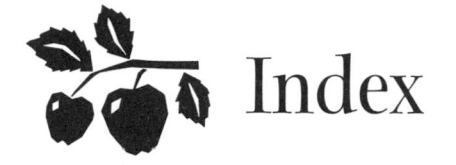 Index

Books of Related Interest

The Slow Down Diet
Eating for Pleasure, Energy and Weight Loss
by Marc David

The Acid–Alkaline Diet for Optimum Health
Restore Your Health by Creating Balance in Your Diet
by Christopher Vasey, N.D.

The Whole Food Bible
How to Select & Prepare Safe, Healthful Foods
by Chris Kilham

Children at Play
Using Waldorf Principles to Foster Childhood Development
by Heidi Britz-Crecelius

Vaccinations: A Thoughtful Parent's Guide
*How to Make Safe, Sensible Decisions about the
Risks, Benefits, and Alternatives*
by Aviva Jill Romm

The Edison Gene
ADHD and the Gift of the Hunter Child
by Thom Hartmann

Walking the World in Wonder
A Children's Herbal
by Ellen Evert Hopman
Illustrations by Jane Allemann

Beyond the Indigo Children
The New Children and the Coming of the Fifth World
by P. M. H. Atwater, L.H.D.

Inner Traditions • Bear & Company
P.O. Box 388
Rochester, VT 05767
1-800-246-8648
www.InnerTraditions.com

Or contact your local bookseller

3 1143 00778 2411